Rheumatologic Manifestations of Endocrine Disease

Guest Editor

JOSEPH A. MARKENSON, MD

RHEUMATIC DISEASE CLINICS OF NORTH AMERICA

www.rheumatic.theclinics.com

November 2010 • Volume 36 • Number 4

SAUNDERS an imprint of ELSEVIER, Inc.

W.B. SAUNDERS COMPANY

A Division of Elsevier Inc.

1600 John F. Kennedy Blvd., Suite 1800 • Philadelphia, PA 19103-2899

http://www.theclinics.com

RHEUMATIC DISEASE CLINICS OF NORTH AMERICA Volume 36, Number 4

November 2010 ISSN 0889-857X, ISBN 13: 978-1-4377-2494-3

Editor: Rachel Glover

Developmental Editor: Natalie Whitted

Photocopying

Single photocopies of single articles may be made for personal use as allowed by national copyright laws. Permission of the Publisher and payment of a fee is required for all other photocopying, including multiple or systematic copying, copying for advertising or promotional purposes, resale, and all forms of document delivery. Special rates are available for educational institutions that wish to make photocopies for non-profit educational classroom use. For information on how to seek permission visit www.elsevier.com/permissions or call: (+44) 1865 843830 (UK)/ (+1) 215 239 3804 (USA).

Derivative Works

Subscribers may reproduce tables of contents or prepare lists of articles including abstracts for internal circulation within their institutions. Permission of the Publisher is required for resale or distribution outside the institution. Permission of the Publisher is required for all other derivative works, including compilations and translations (please consult www.elsevier.com/permissions).

Electronic Storage or Usage

Permission of the Publisher is required to store or use electronically any material contained in this journal, including any article or part of an article (please consult www.elsevier.com/permissions). Except as outlined above, no part of this publication may be reproduced, stored in a retrieval system or transmitted in any form or by any means, electronic, mechanical, photocopying, recording or otherwise, without prior written permission of the Publisher.

Notice

No responsibility is assumed by the Publisher for any injury and/or damage to persons or property as a matter of products liability, negligence or otherwise, or from any use or operation of any methods, products, instructions or ideas contained in the material herein. Because of rapid advances in the medical sciences, in particular, independent verification of diagnoses and drug dosages should be made.

Although all advertising material is expected to conform to ethical (medical) standards, inclusion in this publication does not constitute a guarantee or endorsement of the quality or value of such product or of the claims made of it by its manufacturer.

Rheumatic Disease Clinics of North America (ISSN 0889-857X) is published quarterly by Elsevier Inc., 360 Park Avenue South, New York, NY 10010-1710. Months of issue are February, May, August, and November. Business and editorial offices: 1600 John F. Kennedy Boulevard, Suite 1800, Philadelphia, PA 19103-2899. Periodicals postage paid at New York, NY and additional mailing offices. Subscription prices are USD 282.00 per year for US individuals, USD 501.00 per year for US institutions, USD 139.00 per year for US students and residents, USD 333.00 per year for Canadian individuals, USD 619.00 per year for Canadian institutions, USD 395.00 per year for international individuals, USD 619.00 per year for international institutions, and USD 194.00 per year for Canadian and foreign students/residents. To receive student/resident rate, orders must be accompanied by name of affiliated institution, date of term, and the *signature* of program/residency coordinator on institution letterhead. Orders will be billed at individual rate until proof of status received. Foreign air speed delivery is included in all *Clinics* subscription prices. All prices are subject to change without notice. **POSTMASTER:** Send address changes to *Rheumatic Disease Clinics of North America,* Elsevier Health Sciences Division, Subscription Customer Service, 3251 Riverport Lane, Maryland Heights, MO 63043. **Customer Service: 1-800-654-2452 (US and Canada). From outside of the US and Canada: 314-453-7041. Fax: 314-453-5170. For print support, e-mail: JournalsCustomerService-usa@elsevier.com. For online support, e-mail: JournalsOnline Support-usa@elsevier.com.**

Reprints. For copies of 100 or more of articles in this publication, please contact the Commercial Reprints Department, Elsevier Inc., 360 Park Avenue South, New York, New York, 10010-1710; Tel.: (+1) 212-633-3813, Fax: (+1) 212-462-1935, and E-mail: reprints@elsevier.com.

Rheumatic Disease Clinics of North America is covered in *MEDLINE/PubMed (Index Medicus), Current Contents/Clinical Medicine, Science Citation Index, ISI/BIOMED,* and *EMBASE/Excerpta Medica.*

Printed and bound in the United Kingdom

Transferred to Digital Print 2011

Contributors

GUEST EDITOR

JOSEPH A. MARKENSON, MD, FACP, MACR
Professor of Clinical Medicine, Joan and Sanford Weill Medical College of Cornell University; Attending Physician, Hospital for Special Surgery, New York Presbyterian Hospital, Memorial Sloan-Kettering Cancer Center, New York, New York

AUTHORS

SABEEN ANWAR, MD
Rheumatology Fellow, Division of Rheumatology, Hospital for Special Surgery, New York, New York

ALLAN GIBOFSKY, MD, JD, FACP, FCLM
Professor of Medicine and Public Health, Weill Medical College of Cornell University; Attending Rheumatologist, Division of Rheumatology, Hospital for Special Surgery, New York, New York

Z. HOMÉROVÁ, MD
Fifth Internal Clinic, University Hospital, Bratislava, Slovakia

RICHARD IMRICH, MD, PhD
Professor, Head of Center for Molecular Medicine; Slovak Academy of Sciences, Institute of Experimental Endocrinology, Bratislava, Slovakia

JONATHAN KAY, MD
Professor of Medicine, Director of Clinical Research, Rheumatology Division, Department of Medicine, University of Massachusetts School of Medicine, Worcester, Massachusetts

Z. KILLINGER, MD, PhD
Associate Professor, Head of Osteology, Fifth Internal Clinic, University Hospital, Bratislava, Slovakia

M. KUŽMA, MD
Fifth Internal Clinic, University Hospital, Bratislava, Slovakia

I. LAZÚROVÁ, MD, PhD
Professor, Head of First Department of Internal Medicine, Medical Faculty, Košice, Slovakia

DOROTA LEBIEDZ-ODROBINA, MD
Fellow, Rheumatology Division, Department of Medicine, University of Massachusetts School of Medicine, Worcester, Massachusetts

MICHELLE J. ORMSETH, MD
Rheumatology Fellow, Division of Rheumatology and Immunology, Department of Medicine, Vanderbilt University Medical Center, Vanderbilt University School of Medicine, Nashville, Tennessee

J. PAYER, MD, PhD
Professor, Head of Fifth Internal Clinic, University Hospital, Bratislava, Slovakia

JOZEF ROVENSKÝ, MD, DSc, FRCP
Head of National Institute of Rheumatic Diseases, Piešťany; SS. Cyril and Methodius University in Trnava, Institute the Physiotherapy, Balneology and Therapeutic Rehabilitation, Piešťany, Slovakia

LINDA A. RUSSELL, MD
Assistant Professor of Clinical Medicine, Weill Cornell School of Medicine, Hospital for Special Surgery, New York, New York

LISA R. SAMMARITANO, MD
Associate Professor of Clinical Medicine, Hospital for Special Surgery, Weill Cornell Medical College, New York, New York

H. RALPH SCHUMACHER Jr, MD
Professor, Division of Rheumatology, Department of Medicine, University of Pennsylvania; Veterans Affairs Medical Center, Philadelphia, Pennsylvania

JOHN S. SERGENT, MD
Professor of Medicine, Vice-Chair for Education, Department of Medicine, Vanderbilt University School of Medicine; Vanderbilt University Medical Center, Nashville, Tennessee

HONG YAN WEN, MD
Associate Chief Physician, Shanxi Medical University; Division of Rheumatology, The Second Hospital of Shanxi Medical University, Taiyuan, Shanxi Province, China

LI YUN ZHANG, MD
Professor, Shanxi Medical University; Division of Rheumatology, The Second Hospital of Shanxi Medical University, Taiyuan, Shanxi Province, China

Contents

THE CLINICS ARE NOW AVAILABLE ONLINE!

Access your subscription at:
www.theclinics.com

Preface

Rheumatic Manifestations of Endocrine Disease

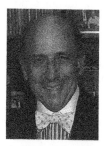

Joseph A. Markenson, MD, MACR
Guest Editor

Rheumatologists in the clinic are faced with different presentations of various musculoskeletal complaints every day. Every new patient encounter requires the differential diagnosis of these complaints. The first task is usually to decide with what disease in Internal Medicine these complaints are associated. The endocrinopathies are a group of illnesses that either present initially or exhibit sometime during the course of the disease as a variety of musculoskeletal complaints. Rheumatic manifestations may often be the initial presentation of an endocrine disorder. Each endocrine disorder may also have its own arthritic complaints, which can present as a definitive rheumatic disease such as calcium pyrophosphate dihydrate deposition disease or as a rheumatic symptom such as diffuse arthralgia. The rheumatologist as well as the primary care physician should be knowledgeable about the ways in which muscles, tendons, ligaments, and joints are affected by diseases of the endocrine system. This issue discusses what is new about these manifestations, as well as the therapeutic options available to treat them.

Each article not only covers older material relating to the occurrence, presence, and pathophysiology of rheumatic complaints in endocrine disease, but also presents new information concerning its prevalence, biology, and genetics. Being aware of the unique presentation and physiology of these complaints will help alert the clinician to an early diagnosis of endocrine disease. In addition, understanding whether certain endocrine disease occurs more often in rheumatologic illness will enable the clinicians to investigate their occurrence early, leading to earlier intervention and resulting in decreased morbidity from these concomitant illnesses.

Each article, where appropriate, reviews the "flip side" and presents material on the occurrence of endocrine disorders in rheumatic disease. In addition, there is a discussion in each article of various autoantibodies seen in rheumatic disease that may be

Rheum Dis Clin N Am 36 (2010) ix–xi
doi:10.1016/j.rdc.2010.10.001   **rheumatic.theclinics.com**
0889-857X/10/$ – see front matter © 2010 Elsevier Inc. All rights reserved.

associated with specific endocrine disorders. The pathophysiology of muscular skeletal complaints in endocrine disease will be discussed. Reports of population as well as genetic studies that address the relationship between endocrine and rheumatologic disease (both of which are often autoimmune) are also presented.

Drs Sabeen Anwar and Allan Gibofsky, in the article on musculoskeletal manifestations of thyroid disease, cover hypo- and hyperthyroidism and their associations with calcium pyrophosphate deposition disease, myopathy, carpal tunnel syndrome, thyroid acropathy, as well as disorders in bone mineral metabolism. In addition, they discuss thyroid disease in patients with known connective tissues disorders as well as the presence and significance of various autoantibodies found in patients with thyroid disorders as well as common connective tissues diseases such as rheumatoid arthritis, Sjogren's syndrome, scleroderma, polymyalgia rheumatica, and systemic lupus erythematosis.

Drs Wen, Schumacher, and Zhang discuss disorders of the parathyroid gland, including musculoskeletal manifestations associated with hypoparathyroidism, such as the "ankylosing spondylitis-like diseases" (DISH). The association of parathyroid disorders with systemic lupus erythematosis and other clinical entities such as corticosteroid treatment and Vitamin D deficiency are also presented. Their article includes a discussion on the "autoimmune pathogenesis" of hyperparathyroidism as well as other manifestations such as neuromyotonia, myopathy, and rhabdomyolyisis. The rest of their article discusses manifestations of hyperparathyroidism such as brown tumors, subperiosteal and/or articular eroisions, deformities, fragility fractures, chondrocalcinosis, gout, myopathy, proximal neuropathy, tendon ruptures, and avulsions.

The article on osteoporosis and osteomalacia by Dr Linda Russell offers a wealth of information discussing the rheumatic consequences of metabolic bone disease, which often is caused by endocrine diseases such as hyperthyroidism, hyperparathyroidism, hypothyroidism, diabetes mellitus, Cushing's disease, and hyperprolactinemia. Additional musculoskeletal manifestations of rickets, osteomalacia, hypophosphatemia, hypomagnesiumia, as well as the role of estrogen and testosterone in maintaining normal bone metabolism are also discussed. Last, Dr Russell updates us on the arthritic syndromes seen in chronic or end-stage renal disease as well as those caused by glucocorticoid use.

Diabetes mellitus is covered by Drs Dorota Lebiedz-Odrobina and Jon Kay, including familiar entities such as diabetic cheiroarthropathy, carpal tunnel syndrome, stenosing flexor tenosynovitis, shoulder adhesive capsulitis, and Duputren's disease. A discussion on the current vascular theories of pathogenesis (resulting from accumulation of advanced glycation end products or AGEs) leading to the various syndromes is reviewed. The role of insulin, growth hormone, and insulin-like growth factor in entities such as diabetic muscle infarction, Charcot neuropathic arthropathy, gout, and pseudo-gout are also discussed.

Musculoskeletal manifestations of disease of the adrenal gland are discussed by Drs Michelle Ormseth and John Sergent. Their article focuses on the similarities between disorders of the adrenal gland and other well-known rheumatic syndromes. In addition, there is an excellent section describing the many symptoms and presentations of adrenal insufficiency so as to help the clinician separate "true" early adrenal insufficiency from other rheumatic disorders.

Acromegaly and its associated arthropathy are described in an article authored by Professor Jozef Rovensky and colleagues. Hypersecretion of growth hormone resulting in excess amounts of insulin-like growth factor-1 is responsible for the increased thickening of connective tissue, resulting in multiple musculoskeletal disorders. The pathophysiology, radiologic changes, and treatment of these disorders are described.

In the article on the hypothalamic-pituitary-adrenal axis (HPA), Drs Richard Imrich and Jozef Rovensky discuss the evidence that the HPA functions as an immune regulator when exposed to high amounts of proinflammatory cytokines (resulting in inappropriately lower levels of cortisol in response to inflammation), possibly contributing to the pathogenesis of inflammatory disease such as rheumatoid arthritis.

Pregnancy, although not generally considered to be an endocrine disorder, nevertheless induces many multisystem changes often similar to endocrine disease, presenting as musculoskeletal complaints. In the last article of this volume Dr Lisa Sammaritano discusses in detail how many complaints including musculoskeletal, dermatologic, hematologic, renal, and neurologic can mimic various symptoms of rheumatic disease. This article covers pathophysiology, presentation, and treatment. Since many new connective tissue diseases can appear during pregnancy (often resulting in worse prognosis), it is imperative to distinguish between pregnancy-induced changes and true autoimmune inflammation, which requires prompt and aggressive treatment.

In summary, this issue presents current data on pathophysiology, pathogenesis, presentation, genetic associations, and treatment of endocrine disease from the perspective of their associated musculoskeletal complaints, which often mimics rheumatic disease. In addition, the association of autoimmune rheumatic disease with various endocrine disorders is also discussed.

Joseph A. Markenson, MD, MACR
Hospital for Special Surgery
Joan and Sanford Weill Medical College of Cornell University
535 East 70th Street
New York, NY 10021, USA

E-mail address:
markensonj@hss.edu

Musculoskeletal Manifestations of Thyroid Disease

Sabeen Anwar, MD[a],*, Allan Gibofsky, MD, JD, FCLM[a,b]

KEYWORDS

• Thyroid • Endocrine • Arthritis

Disorders of the thyroid gland often present with musculoskeletal signs and symptoms. Conversely, rheumatic diseases are frequently associated with autoimmune thyroid disease. This article reviews the common rheumatic presentations of autoimmune thyroid disease as well as discusses the relationship of rheumatic diseases with concurrent thyroid abnormalities. Current viewpoints on the pathophysiologic basis for the disease are reviewed briefly.

HYPOTHYROIDISM

Epidemiology and Clinical Features

The most common cause of primary hypothyroidism in the United States is autoimmunity (Hashimoto thyroiditis). The estimated incidence of Hashimoto thyroiditis is 3.6 per 1000 person-years in women and 0.8 per 1000 person-years in men.[1–3] Other causes include central hypothyroidism (ie, pituitary adenoma or Sheehan syndrome), postpartum thyroiditis, drug-induced causes (ie, lithium), iodine deficiency, and iatrogenesis.

Calcium Pyrophosphate Deposition Disease

Deposition of calcium pyrophosphate dihydrate (CPPD) crystals within the articular cartilage can result in chronic arthropathy (chondrocalcinosis) and/or acute flares of synovitis (pseudogout). Diagnosis is based on the presence of rhomboid intracellular crystals that are weakly positively birefringent under polarized microscopy and/or the presence of intra-articular calcium deposits visualized on radiography.

The association between chondrocalcinosis and hypothyroidism was initially described in a case series of 12 myxedematous patients examined before or within 4 days of thyroid replacement therapy.[4] Musculoskeletal complaints, including joint pain in the hands and knees, were observed. Among the 12 patients, 9 had knee

[a] Division of Rheumatology, Hospital for Special Surgery, 535 East 70th Street, New York, NY 10021, USA
[b] Department of Medicine and Public Health, Weill Medical College of Cornell University, 1300 York Avenue, New York, NY 10065, USA
* Corresponding author.
E-mail address: sabeenanwar@gmail.com

Rheum Dis Clin N Am 36 (2010) 637–646
doi:10.1016/j.rdc.2010.09.001
0889-857X/10/$ – see front matter © 2010 Published by Elsevier Inc.

rheumatic.theclinics.com

effusions that were typically bilateral. The joint effusions had a characteristically high viscosity and were difficult to ascertain by routine physical examination, often confused for synovial thickening. In addition, synovitis of the wrists, metacarpal joints, and flexor tendon sheaths was noted. Synovial fluid analysis demonstrated the presence of intra- and extracellular positively birefringent crystals consistent with CPPD. However, the presence of chondrocalcinosis was distinguished from acute attacks of pseudogout, which was not observed in most patients.

Subsequently, 4 surveys examining the prevalence of knee chondrocalcinosis among hypothyroid patients compared with healthy patients failed to demonstrate a statistically significant risk association.[5–8] However, these studies were likely underpowered to detect significant change. A meta-analysis of these studies produced an odds ratio of 1.94 suggesting a small association between the 2 disorders.

In addition to hypothyroidism, CPPD is associated with other metabolic disorders such as hyperparathyroidism, hypomagnesemia, hypophosphatasia, hemachromatosis, gout, Wilson disease, acromegaly, and familial hypocalciuric hypercalcemia. The mechanism whereby an altered metabolic milieu in thyroid disease could contribute to the influx of calcium deposits into the joint is not well understood. Inorganic pyrophosphate levels in synovial fluid have been measured to be lower in hypothyroid patients than normal patients as well as in other disease states associated with CPPD, which does not support the association between the 2 diseases.[9]

Hypothyroid Myopathy

Muscle symptoms may manifest in 25% to 79% of adult patients with hypothyroidism.[10,11] The symptoms often reported by patients are pain, cramps, stiffness, easy fatigability, and weakness. Physical examination findings may include muscle hypertrophy, proximal muscle weakness, and delayed relaxation phase of deep tendon reflexes.[12] Mounding is a sustained focal contraction of skeletal muscles on striking with a reflex hammer and is a nonspecific finding in hypothyroid myopathy. Mounding may be related, in part, to delayed reuptake of released calcium ion by the sarcoplasmic reticulum.[13]

Hoffman syndrome is a rare clinical disorder of severe hypothyroid myopathy, which manifests with severe muscle stiffness, increased muscle mass (pseudohypertrophy), variable muscle weakness along with elevated levels of creatine kinase (CK).[14] Kocher-Debré-Sémélaigne syndrome is a disorder of infancy associated with the features of cretinism (short stature, enlarged tongue, neurologic impairment in the setting of maternal iodine deficiency) and muscular pseudohypertrophy. Kocher's original description in 1892 in a young man with cretinism first shed light on the relationship between the thyroid and skeletal muscles. As such, this syndrome is rarely encountered in the era of newborn screening for thyroid disease. There are no painful muscle spasms as in Hoffman syndrome. Muscle enzyme levels are typically elevated, and there is type I fiber atrophy on muscle biopsy.[15,16]

Serum muscle enzyme levels are frequently elevated in patients with hypothyroid myopathy and are elevated in up to 90% of asymptomatic patients.[11,17,18] These enzymes include CK, myoglobin, and lactate dehydrogenase.[19] Although this increase is typically mild (CK<1000 IU/L), numerous reports of a polymyositis-like illness or rhabdomyolysis with dramatic elevations in CK levels do exist in the literature.[20,21] Correlation between elevated CK levels and thyrotropin-stimulating hormone (TSH) levels has been observed but not with a degree of weakness.[11,22]

Diagnosis may be supported by electromyography (EMG), which is often normal but helps in distinguishing hypothyroid myopathy from other myopathies. Reported features include repetitive positive waves, increased insertional activity, and fibrillations.[23–25] On muscle biopsy, there is characteristic atrophy of type II muscle fibers, with relative hypertrophy in type I muscle fibers. Other nonspecific findings include an increase in the percentage of type I fibers, presence of internalized nuclei, and corelike structures.[12,22,26–28] In most cases of hypothyroid myopathy, symptoms resolve within approximately 6 months of therapy with supplemental thyroxine.[11,29]

Several explanations have been postulated for the effect of thyroid hormones on skeletal muscle tissues. Changes in fiber type from fast to slow contribute to the delayed contraction and relaxation. Alteration in myosin heavy chain gene forms may lead to changes in energy use by the muscle.[30] Impaired glycogenolysis may also be contributory.

Carpal Tunnel Syndrome

Carpal tunnel syndrome (CTS) is an increasingly common neuromuscular disorder with an estimated prevalence of 3.8% in the general population.[31] However, practitioners should remain vigilant of its association with hypothyroidism, diabetes mellitus, and inflammatory disorders. One systematic review of 4908 patients with CTS found a pooled odds ratio of 1.4 (95% CI, 1.0–2.0) for the prevalence of concomitant hypothyroidism compared with healthy controls.[11,32]

There are 9 flexor tendons and the median nerve coursing through the carpal tunnel ligament on the volar aspect of the wrist. When this compartment is compressed, patients commonly experience pain or paresthesias in the distribution of the median nerve. These symptoms may be worse at night or with flexion at the wrist. There may be weakness or atrophy of the thenar muscles in prolonged cases. Physical maneuvers such as Tinel and Phalen signs or 2-point discrimination may be useful in the diagnosis of CTS.[33] Bilateral CTS has been reported in hypothyroidism.[34] The mechanism for compression is thought to be secondary to the accumulation of glycosaminoglycans (GAGs) within the surrounding tissues.[35]

Electrodiagnostic studies are the gold standard for diagnosing CTS. Therapy may include both medical and surgical options such as wrist splinting, corticosteroid injection, or carpal tunnel release for severe cases. Treatment of underlying hypothyroidism has been shown to ameliorate the course of CTS in most studies,[34,36] although one article reported ongoing clinical and electrodiagnostic manifestations in hypothyroid patients once they returned to a euthyroid state.[37]

HYPERTHYROIDISM
Epidemiology and Clinical Features

Hyperthyroidism may be secondary to a variety of causes including autoimmune, infectious, drug-induced, or iatrogenic. Graves disease, the most common cause of hyperthyroidism worldwide, has an estimated incidence of 100 to 200 cases per annum,[2,3] with an increased susceptibility in women.

Myopathy

Hyperthyroid myopathy has a similar presentation as hypothyroidism, with proximal muscle manifesting early in the disease course in up to 67% of patients in 1 study. Other complaints, including myalgia or fatigability, are less frequently reported. In contrast with hypothyroidism, serum CK levels are typically normal and myopathic findings on EMG were rare (10% of patients). Symptoms of weakness resolve with a mean 3.6 months of therapy for hyperthyroidism.[11] Muscle biopsy, if ever performed, demonstrates fiber atrophy and fat infiltration.[38]

Pretibial Myxedema

Infiltrative dermopathy, or pretibial myxedema, is a rare manifestation of Graves disease and is a marker for Graves ophthalmopathy (seen in 97% of patients).[39] Clinically, the skin of the lower extremities is typically affected with induration, nonpitting edema, and a peau d'orange appearance in the pretibial areas. The lesions may range in size and are not painful but may be itchy or unsightly. Biopsy of the lesions shows the presence of GAGs and the damage to collagen and elastin fibers.[40] Treatment with topical corticosteroids is effective in 50% of patients unless the lesions are chronic or severe.[41]

It is postulated that GAGs released by skin fibroblasts accumulate in the dermis and subcutis. The triggering event is unknown but may be related to autoantibody stimulation of a cross-reacting thyroid antigen. Another theory relates to aberrant production or degradation of GAGs mediated by prostaglandins.[42] In addition, analysis of the T-cell receptor variable gene region of the involved skin demonstrates a restricted repertoire, suggesting a role for antigen-specific T cells in the development of dermopathy.[43]

Thyroid acropachy, or new periosteal bone formation, leading to clubbing of the fingers and toes may also be seen. Plain radiographs show periosteal reaction. These findings are associated with Graves ophthalmopathy and dermatopathy and may have a higher prevalence in smokers.[44,45]

Altered Bone Metabolism

Perhaps the most serious musculoskeletal consequence of untreated hyperthyroidism is ongoing rapid bone turnover leading to a decline in bone mineral density (BMD). Excess thyroxine secretion leads to increased bone resorption time with a decrease in mineralization time, leading to net resorptive effect.[46] This effect is likely mediated by indirect osteoblast activation of osteoclasts.[47] Serum calcium levels are increased in hyperthyroidism because of increased bone resorption and similarly hypercalciuria is also present leading to a negative calcium balance.[48] In addition, concentration of bone turnover markers, including serum alkaline phosphatase, osteocalcin, and urinary hydroxyproline, is increased. The amount of both cortical and trabecular bone is decreased.[49,50]

Comparison of bone densitometry scores of patients with active hyperthyroidism, treated euthyroid patients, and controls highlighted a mean z score ranging from −0.79 to −0.92 (based on the site) in the untreated patients. Euthyroid patients had z scores ranging from −0.23 to −0.74, which are still less than age- and sex-adjusted controls with a z score ranging from 0.09 to 0.36.[51] One long-term study that followed up patients with hyperthyroidism who achieved prolonged euthyroid state demonstrated an increase in lumbar BMD at 5 years suggesting a reversibility of this effect. High triiodothyronine levels during illness positively correlated with a subsequent improvement in BMD.[52] The risk of hip fracture was elevated in a meta-analysis of 5 studies of hyperthyroid patients.[53]

These data suggest that close monitoring of BMD in hyperthyroid patients alongside treatment is essential in preventing osteoporosis. Maintenance of adequate levels of calcium and vitamin D is important. Treatment with alendronate and methimazole may be better than methimazole alone for improvement of BMD.[54]

THYROID DISEASE IN PATIENTS WITH CONNECTIVE TISSUE DISORDERS
Autoantibodies

In autoimmune thyroid disease, several autoantibodies play a role in the disease pathogenesis. In Graves disease, stimulatory autoantibodies to TSH receptor (TSHR Abs) cause the development of illness via their stimulatory action on cyclic AMP leading to thyroxine secretion.[55] TSHR Abs are also highly specific for Graves disease. However, antithyroid peroxidase and antithyroglobulin are present in both Hashimoto and Graves disease and are increasingly recognized in systemic autoimmune illnesses. In one retrospective review of 300 cases of systemic lupus erythematosus (SLE), 14% of patients had antithyroid antibodies and 5.7% had hypothyroidism (compared with a baseline prevalence of 1.7%).[56] The upregulation of polyclonal autoantibodies to thyroid is reflective of the amplified humoral immune response in SLE.

Conversely, antinuclear antibody to the nucleus and single-stranded DNA has been observed in 26% and 34%, respectively, of patients with autoimmune thyroid disease (Graves disease or Hashimoto thyroiditis), significantly higher than age-matched healthy controls in the absence of any identifiable connective tissue disorder. These patients lacked the presence of anti–double-stranded DNA, extractable nuclear antigen, anti–SS-A and anti–SS-B antibodies, or rheumatoid factor.[57] It should be noted that 1 subgroup of hypothyroid mothers with positive Ro antibodies had an increased incidence for delivering a child with complete congenital heart block.[58]

Autoimmune Diseases

A large multicenter cross-sectional study in the United Kingdom sought to identify the prevalence and relative risk of systemic autoimmune diseases in patients with preexisting autoimmune thyroid disease. Furthermore, familial clustering of autoimmune diseases was evaluated. A dramatic increase of a concomitant autoimmune disease in 9.67% of patients with Graves disease and 14.3% with Hashimoto thyroiditis was noted. The estimated relative risk exceeded 10-fold for several diseases, including SLE, vitiligo, pernicious anemia, and celiac disease.[59]

In SLE, antithyroid antibodies (antithyroglobulin and antimicrosomal) are present in 14% of patients, increasing to 68% in the subgroup with thyroid disease. In patients with thyroid disease diagnosed after SLE, antithyroid antibodies were present before the development of thyroid disease, suggesting a causal relationship.[56] A genetic linkage study of 35 families with cases of concomitant SLE and autoimmune thyroid disease, a susceptibility gene at 5q14.3-q15 was identified. This result highlights a potential genetic link between the 2 diseases, but further studies are needed.[60]

Rheumatoid arthritis (RA) has been associated with an increased prevalence of both antithyroid antibodies[61,62] and autoimmune thyroid disease, ranging from 16% to 30% in cases versus 9% to 10% in controls.[63,64] One study demonstrated a four-fold risk of cardiovascular diseases in female RA patients with clinical hypothyroidism independent of other risk factor such as hypertension, smoking, age, gender and diabetes. These findings show the importance of the dyslipidemia associated with hypothyroidism.[65] Among the seronegative spondyloarthropathies, psoriatic arthritis has also been linked with an autoimmune thyroid disease, with possibly a predilection for patients with polyarticular involvement and longer disease duration.[66]

The association of thyroid disorders with Sjögren syndrome is not entirely clear because of the studies that may have been confounded by additional risk factors such as female gender or advancing age, which also confer additional risk for thyroid disease. One retrospective study reported an increased percentage of Hashimoto thyroiditis at a rate of 6.26% in a Hungarian cohort; however, there was no association found with Graves disease.[67] Likewise, another study of 114 patients demonstrated a rate of 14% for hypothyroidism and 1.8% for Graves disease in patients with Sjögren syndrome.[68] Furthermore, the sicca complaints independent of the diagnosis of Sjögren syndrome were observed in up to 27% of patients with thyroid disease.[69]

In a relatively small study of 66 patients with juvenile idiopathic arthritis, mean TSH levels were above normal in 12.0% of the patients compared with 3.4% controls and the level of antithyroid autoantibodies was elevated as well.[70]

The association between scleroderma and thyroid disease is unique in that the disease may result in fibrosis of the thyroid gland in the absence of a lymphocytic infiltrate.[5] Fewer than half of the patients have antithyroid antibodies. In patients with mixed connective tissue disease, antithyroid antibodies are present in 25% and hypothyroidism in less than 20%.[71,72]

In patients with autoimmune thyroid disease, one study noted the prevalence of polymyalgia rheumatica/giant cell arteritis (PMR/GCA) as 2.8%. All cases occurred in women older than 60 years. A comparative group of 150 women from a cardiac clinic had no cases of PMR/GCA. Conversely, some studies have shown an increased rate of autoimmune thyroid disease in patients with PMR/GCA.[73,74] The largest of these studies was conducted in 367 patients, with 4.9% of patients having overt hypothyroidism. It should be noted that although the findings were statistically significant, the control population of 84 normal participants had an unusually low rate of disease.[74] Also, similarities between the 2 disease states (myalgias, proximal muscle symptoms) may actually be confounding. In addition, the 2 studies failed to show an association between PMR/GCA.[75,76]

Fibromyalgia is another rheumatic disorder that has been associated with autoimmune thyroid disease. One study cited as high as 20% to 24% prevalence of antithyroid antibodies in patients with fibromyalgia without evidence of overt thyroid disease, with a particular increase among older and postmenopausal patients.[77] Another study evaluated the response of patients with fibromyalgia to intravenous injection of TRH and found a diminished secretion of thyroid hormones after 2 hours in the patients with the disease as compared with healthy donors.[78]

SUMMARY

The relationship between thyroid disorders and rheumatic diseases is significant. Thyroid diseases not only emulate rheumatic disease with findings such as myopathy or arthropathy but also frequently manifest with primary rheumatologic complaints that the practitioner should be wary of, such as calcium pyrophosphate deposition disease. There is increasing recognition of the prevalence of autoimmune thyroid diseases in patients with connective tissue disorder, highlighting a common mechanism for the disease pathogenesis, which requires further inquiry.

REFERENCES

1. Aoki Y, Belin RM, Clickner R, et al. Serum TSH and total T4 in the United States population and their association with participant characteristics: National Health and Nutrition Examination Survey (NHANES 1999–2002). Thyroid 2007;17(12):1211–23.
2. Tunbridge WM, Evered DC, Hall R, et al. The spectrum of thyroid disease in a community: the Whickham survey. Clin Endocrinol (Oxf) 1977;7(6):481–93.
3. Vanderpump MP, Tunbridge WM, French JM, et al. The incidence of thyroid disorders in the community: a twenty-year follow-up of the Whickham Survey. Clin Endocrinol (Oxf) 1995;43(1):55–68.
4. Dorwart BB, Schumacher HR. Joint effusions, chondrocalcinosis and other rheumatic manifestations in hypothyroidism. A clinicopathologic study. Am J Med 1975;59(6):780–90.
5. Gordon TP, Smith M, Ebert B, et al. Articular chondrocalcinosis in a hospital population: an Australian experience. Aust N Z J Med 1984;14(5):655–9.

6. Komatireddy GR, Ellman MH, Brown NL. Lack of association between hypothyroidism and chondrocalcinosis. J Rheumatol 1989;16(6):807–8.
7. Job-Deslandre C, Menkes CJ, Guinot M, et al. Does hypothyroidism increase the prevalence of chondrocalcinosis? Br J Rheumatol 1993;32(3):197–8.
8. Jones AC, Chuck AJ, Arie EA, et al. Diseases associated with calcium pyrophosphate deposition disease. Semin Arthritis Rheum 1992;22(3):188–202.
9. Doherty M, Chuck A, Hoskin D, et al. Inorganic pyrophosphate in metabolic diseases predisposing to calcium pyrophosphate dihydrate crystal deposition. Arthritis Rheum 1991;34(10):1297–303.
10. Hartl E, Finsterer J, Grossegger C, et al. Relationship between thyroid function and skeletal muscle in subclinical and overt hypothyroidism. Endocrinologist 2001;11:217–21.
11. Duyff RF, Van den Bosch J, Laman DM, et al. Neuromuscular findings in thyroid dysfunction: a prospective clinical and electrodiagnostic study. J Neurol Neurosurg Psychiatr 2000;68(6):750–5.
12. Cruz MW, Tendrich M, Vaisman M, et al. Electroneuromyography and neuromuscular findings in 16 primary hypothyroidism patients. Arq Neuropsiquiatr 1996;54(1):12–8.
13. Mizusawa H, Takagi A, Nonaka I, et al. Muscular abnormalities in experimental hypothyroidism of rats with special reference to the mounding phenomenon. Exp Neurol 1984;85(3):480–92.
14. Klein I, Parker M, Shebert R, et al. Hypothyroidism presenting as muscle stiffness and pseudohypertrophy: Hoffmann's syndrome. Am J Med 1981;70(4):891–4.
15. Tullu MS, Udgirkar VS, Muranjan MN, et al. Kocher-Debre-Semelaigne syndrome: hypothyroidism with muscle pseudohypertrophy. Indian J Pediatr 2003;70(8):671–3.
16. Spiro AJ, Hirano A, Beilin RL, et al. Cretinism with muscular hypertrophy (Kocher-Debré-Sémélaigne syndrome). Histochemical and ultrastructural study of skeletal muscle. Arch Neurol 1970;23(4):340–9.
17. Graig FA, Ross G. Serum creatine-phosphokinase in thyroid disease. Metabolism 1963;12:57–9.
18. Griffiths PD. Serum enzymes in diseases of the thyroid gland. J Clin Pathol 1965;18(5):660–3.
19. Giampietro O, Clerico A, Buzzigoli G, et al. Detection of hypothyroid myopathy by measurement of various serum muscle markers—myoglobin, creatine kinase, lactate dehydrogenase and their isoenzymes. Correlations with thyroid hormone levels (free and total) and clinical usefulness. Horm Res 1984;19(4):232–42.
20. Madariaga MG. Polymyositis-like syndrome in hypothyroidism: review of cases reported over the past twenty-five years. Thyroid 2002;12(4):331–6.
21. Scott KR, Simmons Z, Boyer PJ. Hypothyroid myopathy with a strikingly elevated serum creatine kinase level. Muscle Nerve 2002;26(1):141–4.
22. McKeran RO, Ward P, Slavin G, et al. Central nuclear counts in muscle fibres before and during treatment in hypothyroid myopathy. J Clin Pathol 1979;32(3):229–33.
23. Scarpalezos S, Lygidakis C, Papageorgiou C, et al. Neural and muscular manifestations of hypothyroidism. Arch Neurol 1973;29(3):140–4.
24. Klein I, Levey GS. Unusual manifestations of hypothyroidism [review]. Arch Intern Med 1984;144(1):123–8.
25. Norris FH Jr, Panner BJ. Hypothyroid myopathy. Clinical, electromyographical, and ultrastructural observations. Arch Neurol 1966;14(6):574–89.

26. Khaleeli AA, Griffith DG, Edwards RH. The clinical presentation of hypothyroid myopathy and its relationship to abnormalities in structure and function of skeletal muscle. Clin Endocrinol (Oxf) 1983;19(3):365–76.

27. Evans RM, Watanabe I, Singer PA. Central changes in hypothyroid myopathy: a case report. Muscle Nerve 1990;13(10):952–6.

28. Ono S, Inouye K, Mannen T. Myopathology of hypothyroid myopathy. Some new observations. J Neurol Sci 1987;77(2–3):237–48.

29. Mastaglia FL, Ojeda VJ, Sarnat HB, et al. Myopathies associated with hypothyroidism: a review based upon 13 cases. Aust N Z J Med 1988;18(6):799–806.

30. Caiozzo VJ, Baker MJ, Baldwin KM. Novel transitions in MHC isoforms: separate and combined effects of thyroid hormone and mechanical unloading. J Appl Physiol 1998;85(6):2237–48.

31. Atroshi I, Gummesson C, Johnsson R, et al. Prevalence of carpal tunnel syndrome in a general population. JAMA 1999;282(2):153–8.

32. van Dijk MA, Reitsma JB, Fischer JC, et al. Indications for requesting laboratory tests for concurrent diseases in patients with carpal tunnel syndrome: a systematic review. Clin Chem 2003;49(9):1437–44.

33. Katz JN, Larson MG, Sabra A, et al. The carpal tunnel syndrome: diagnostic utility of the history and physical examination findings. Ann Intern Med 1990;112(5):321–7.

34. Chisholm JC Jr. Hypothyroidism: a rare cause of the bilateral carpal tunnel syndrome–a case report and a review of the literature. J Natl Med Assoc 1981; 73(11):1082–5.

35. Purnell DC, Daly DD, Lipscomb PR. Carpal-tunnel syndrome associated with myxedema. Arch Intern Med 1961;108:751–6.

36. Kececi H, Degirmenci Y. Hormone replacement therapy in hypothyroidism and nerve conduction study. Neurophysiol Clin 2006;36(2):79–83.

37. Palumbo CF, Szabo RM, Olmsted SL. The effects of hypothyroidism and thyroid replacement on the development of carpal tunnel syndrome. J Hand Surg Am 2000;25(4):734–9.

38. Ramsay ID. Muscle dysfunction in hyperthyroidism. Lancet 1966;2(7470):931–4.

39. Fatourechi V, Pajouhi M, Fransway AF. Dermopathy of Graves disease (pretibial myxedema). Review of 150 cases. Medicine (Baltimore) 1994;73(1):1–7.

40. Kriss JP. Pathogenesis and treatment of pretibial myxedema. Endocrinol Metab Clin North Am 1987;16(2):409–15.

41. Schwartz KM, Fatourechi V, Ahmed DD, et al. Dermopathy of Graves' disease (pretibial myxedema): long-term outcome. J Clin Endocrinol Metab 2002;87(2): 438–46.

42. Komosińska-Vassev K, Winsz-Szczotka K, Olczyk K, et al. Alterations in serum glycosaminoglycan profiles in Graves' patients. Clin Chem Lab Med 2006; 44(5):582–8.

43. Heufelder AE, Bahn RS, Scriba PC. Analysis of T cell antigen receptor variable region gene usage in patients with thyroid-related pretibial dermopathy. J Invest Dermatol 1995;105(3):372–8.

44. Nixon DW, Samols E. Acral changes in thyroid disorders. N Engl J Med 1971; 284(20):1158–9.

45. Fatourechi V, Ahmed DD, Schwartz KM. Thyroid acropachy: report of 40 patients treated at a single institution in a 26-year period. J Clin Endocrinol Metab 2002; 87(12):5435–41.

46. Mosekilde L, Melsen F. A tetracycline-based histomorphometric evaluation of bone resorption and bone turnover in hyperthyroidism and hyperparathyroidism. Acta Med Scand 1978;204(1–2):97–102.

47. Britto JM, Fenton AJ, Holloway WR, et al. Osteoblasts mediate thyroid hormone stimulation of osteoclastic bone resorption. Endocrinology 1994;134(1):169–76.
48. Daly JG, Greenwood RM, Himsworth RL. Serum calcium concentration in hyperthyroidism at diagnosis and after treatment. Clin Endocrinol (Oxf) 1983;19(3):397–404.
49. Toh SH, Claunch BC, Brown PH. Effect of hyperthyroidism and its treatment on bone mineral content. Arch Intern Med 1985;145(5):883–6.
50. Fraser SA, Anderson JB, Smith DA, et al. Osteoporosis and fractures following thyrotoxicosis. Lancet 1971;1(7707):981–3.
51. Jódar E, Muñoz-Torres M, Escobar-Jiménez F, et al. Bone loss in hyperthyroid patients and in former hyperthyroid patients controlled on medical therapy: influence of aetiology and menopause. Clin Endocrinol (Oxf) 1997;47(3):279–85.
52. Rosen CJ, Adler RA. Longitudinal changes in lumbar bone density among thyrotoxic patients after attainment of euthyroidism. J Clin Endocrinol Metab 1992;75(6):1531–4.
53. Vestergaard P, Mosekilde L. Hyperthyroidism, bone mineral, and fracture risk– a meta-analysis. Thyroid 2003;13(6):585–93.
54. Lupoli G, Nuzzo V, Di Carlo C, et al. Effects of alendronate on bone loss in pre- and postmenopausal hyperthyroid women treated with methimazole. Gynecol Endocrinol 1996;10(5):343–8.
55. Laurent E, Mockel J, Van Sande J, et al. Dual activation by thyrotropin of the phospholipase C and cyclic AMP cascades in human thyroid. Mol Cell Endocrinol 1987;52(3):273–8.
56. Pyne D, Isenberg DA. Autoimmune thyroid disease in systemic lupus erythematosus. Ann Rheum Dis 2002;61(1):70–2.
57. Morita S, Arima T, Matsuda M. Prevalence of nonthyroid specific autoantibodies in autoimmune thyroid diseases. J Clin Endocrinol Metab 1995;80(4):1203–6.
58. Spence D, Hornberger L, Hamilton R, et al. Increased risk of complete congenital heart block in infants born to women with hypothyroidism and anti-Ro and/or anti-La antibodies. J Rheumatol 2006;33(1):167–70.
59. Boelaert K, Newby PR, Simmonds MJ, et al. Prevalence and relative risk of other autoimmune diseases in subjects with autoimmune thyroid disease. Am J Med 2010;123(2):183, e1–9.
60. Namjou B, Kelly JA, Kilpatrick J, et al. Linkage at 5q14.3-15 in multiplex systemic lupus erythematosus pedigrees stratified by autoimmune thyroid disease. Arthritis Rheum 2005;52(11):3646–50.
61. Magnus JH, Birketvedt T, Haga HJ. A prospective evaluation of antithyroid antibody prevalence in 100 patients with rheumatoid arthritis. Scand J Rheumatol 1995;24(3):180–2.
62. Atzeni F, Doria A, Ghirardello A, et al. Anti-thyroid antibodies and thyroid dysfunction in rheumatoid arthritis: prevalence and clinical value. Autoimmunity 2008;41(1):111–5.
63. Shiroky JB, Cohen M, Ballachey ML, et al. Thyroid dysfunction in rheumatoid arthritis: a controlled prospective survey. Ann Rheum Dis 1993;52(6):454–6.
64. Przygodzka M, Filipowicz-Sosnowska A. Prevalence of thyroid diseases and antithyroid antibodies in women with rheumatoid arthritis. Pol Arch Med Wewn 2009;119(1–2):39–43.
65. Raterman HG, Van Halm VP, Voskuyl AE, et al. Rheumatoid arthritis is associated with a high prevalence of hypothyroidism that amplifies its cardiovascular risk. Ann Rheum Dis 2008;67(2):229–32.

66. Antonelli A, Delle Sedie A, Fallahi P, et al. High prevalence of thyroid autoimmunity and hypothyroidism in patients with psoriatic arthritis. J Rheumatol 2006; 33(10):2026–8.
67. Zeher M, Horvath IF, Szanto A, et al. Autoimmune thyroid diseases in a large group of Hungarian patients with primary Sjögren's syndrome. Thyroid 2009; 19(1):39–45.
68. Lazarus MN, Isenberg DA. Development of additional autoimmune diseases in a population of patients with primary Sjögren's syndrome. Ann Rheum Dis 2005;64(7):1062–4.
69. Hansen BU, Ericsson UB, Henricsson V, et al. Autoimmune thyroiditis and primary Sjögren's syndrome: clinical and laboratory evidence of the coexistence of the two diseases. Clin Exp Rheumatol 1991;9(2):137–41.
70. Harel L, Prais D, Uziel Y, et al. Increased prevalence of antithyroid antibodies and subclinical hypothyroidism in children with juvenile idiopathic arthritis. J Rheumatol 2006;33(1):164–6.
71. Kahl LE, Medsger TA Jr, Klein I. Prospective evaluation of thyroid function in patients with systemic sclerosis (scleroderma). J Rheumatol 1986;13(1):103–7.
72. Hämeenkorpi R, Hakala M, Ruuska P, et al. Thyroid disorder in patients with mixed connective tissue disease. J Rheumatol 1993;20(3):602–3.
73. Bowness P, Shotliff K, Middlemiss A, et al. Prevalence of hypothyroidism in patients with polymyalgia rheumatica and giant cell arteritis. Br J Rheumatol 1991;30(5):349–51.
74. Wiseman P, Stewart K, Rai GS. Hypothyroidism in polymyalgia rheumatica and giant cell arteritis. BMJ 1989;298(6674):647–8.
75. Barrier JH, Abram M, Brisseau JM, et al. Autoimmune thyroid disease, thyroid antibodies and giant cell arteritis: the supposed correlation appears fortuitous. J Rheumatol 1992;19(11):1733–4.
76. Dasgupta B, Grundy E, Stainer E. Hypothyroidism in polymyalgia rheumatica and giant cell arteritis: lack of any association. BMJ 1990;301(6743):96–7.
77. Pamuk ON, Cakir N. The frequency of thyroid antibodies in fibromyalgia patients and their relationship with symptoms. Clin Rheumatol 2007;26(1):55–9.
78. Neeck G, Riedel W. Thyroid function in patients with fibromyalgia syndrome. J Rheumatol 1992;19(7):1120–2.

Parathyroid Disease

Hong Yan Wen, MD[a,b], H. Ralph Schumacher Jr, MD[c],
Li Yun Zhang, MD[a,b],*

KEYWORDS

- Hypocalcemia • Hypercalcemia • Myopathy • Gout
- Pseudogout • Bone disease

Parathyroid diseases can be associated with important musculoskeletal problems. These problems vary from well-recognized bone diseases to rare complications. This review addresses the joint, bone, and soft-tissue problems that can occur in patients with hyperparathyroidism and hypoparathyroidism. Parathyroid hormone (PTH) works in conjunction with vitamin D to regulate the total body calcium. PTH has dual actions, both anabolic and catabolic, on the skeleton. PTH provides a powerful mechanism for controlling extracellular calcium and phosphate concentrations. Moreover, it exerts a potent influence in the conversion of 25-hydroxycholecalciferol to 1,25-dihydroxycholecalciferol in the proximal tubules of the kidneys.

HYPOPARATHYROIDISM

The absence of PTH or resistance to PTH by the target organs, especially bones and kidneys, results in low serum ionized calcium, high serum phosphate, and decreased 1,25-dihydroxycholecalciferol.[1] Such a low serum calcium level affects the central and peripheral nervous system, skeletal muscles, and myocardium and can be manifested by neuromuscular irritability, depression, neuropsychiatric manifestations, convulsions, paresthesias, muscle cramps, tetany, prolonged QT intervals, and cardiac failure.

Deficient PTH secretion has postsurgical or idiopathic causes. Idiopathic causes are further categorized into congenital or acquired. Congenital hypoparathyroidism is a condition in which the person is born without parathyroid tissue. Patients usually have no family history of the disease. The acquired form of the disease typically arises because the immune system developed antibodies against the parathyroid tissues. In

Funding support: none.
The authors have nothing to disclose.
[a] Shanxi Medical University, 86# South Xinjian, Shanxi Province, China
[b] Division of Rheumatology, The Second Hospital of Shanxi Medical University, 382# Wuyi Road, Taiyuan, Shanxi Province 030001, China
[c] Division of Rheumatology, Department of Medicine, University of Pennsylvania VA Medical Center, PA, USA
* Corresponding author. Division of Rheumatology, The Second Hospital of Shanxi Medical University, 382# Wuyi Road, Taiyuan, Shanxi Province 030001, China.
E-mail address: Zhangly2006@sina.com

response to this, the parathyroid stops synthesizing and secreting PTH. The authors discuss this acquired form of the disease in this article.

Hypoparathyroidism usually starts insidiously, with slowly increasing episodic symptoms dominated by increased musculoskeletal irritability. The main symptoms, such as muscle cramps, stiffness, tetany, and paresthesias, may enter the differential diagnosis of the rheumatic diseases. There may be subcutaneous nodules caused by soft-tissue calcification. Although hypoparathyroidism is not uncommon, the diagnosis is often missed because of its unusual clinical manifestations. The mechanism underlying these skeletal changes in hypoparathyroidism is not well defined. The associated musculoskeletal syndromes are subsequently described.

Ankylosing Spondylitis-like Diseases or Diffuse Idiopathic Skeletal Hyperostosis

The skeletal abnormalities of hypoparathyroidism are caused by calcification, which can simulate ankylosing spondylitis with clinical signs, including morning stiffness, gait, and posture.[2–7] Sacroiliitis is not expected, although it is the earliest manifestation in most patients with ankylosing spondylitis. There may be sacroiliac sclerosis, but not erosions. The patterns of syndesmophytes in patients with hypoparathyroidism can resemble those of ankylosing spondylitis with origin from the vertebral margin and preserved disc space, but more often there is also involvement of the posterior paraspinal ligament.[3,6] The syndesmophytes reported have been predominantly present in the thoracic and upper lumbar region. Bone density is generally increased in hypoparathyroidism.[3] The syndesmophytes observed have been different from osteophytes of degenerative axial arthritis in that the latter osteophytes spread horizontally before curving up and there is reduction in the disc space. In some cases, these spinal changes are associated with bony proliferation about the pelvis, hip, and long bones, and soft-tissue and tendon calcifications.[7] Although sacroiliac joints are generally spared, periarticular ossification has been recorded in this location. The preservation of sacroiliac joints, HLA B-27 negativity, as well as less significant involvement of the anterior intervertebral ligament does not fit with the diagnosis of ankylosing spondylitis. The pain does not disappear despite taking immunosuppressive agents and nonsteroidal antiinflammatory drugs, but many resolve completely with treatment by calcitriol.[8]

Serum calcium may need to be included in the diagnostic work-up of patients with inflammatory back pain, especially if they present with atypical features as previously described. It is important to differentiate hypoparathyroid-related spondylitis from ankylosing spondylitis because the management for the two disorders is different. In fact, some of the drugs used for ankylosing spondylitis, such as bisphosphonates, may worsen hypocalcemia.

The mechanism underlying these skeletal changes in hypoparathyroidism is not well defined. Decreased intestinal calcium absorption caused by a defect in the action of 1,25-dihydroxyvitamin D (1,25[OH] 2D) has been suggested to play a role in a controlled study of paravertebral ligamentous ossification.[9]

Spinal changes in hypoparathyroidism have also been described to be similar to those in diffuse idiopathic skeletal hyperostosis (DISH) (**Fig. 1**), which is characterized by ossification of the anterior longitudinal ligament, of the spine, and various extraspinal ligaments, but is rarely reported before the 50 years of age. Okazaki and colleagues[10] suggested that the ossifying diathesis of paravertebral ligaments, which is the origin of DISH, might be initiated or aggravated by hypoparathyroidism.

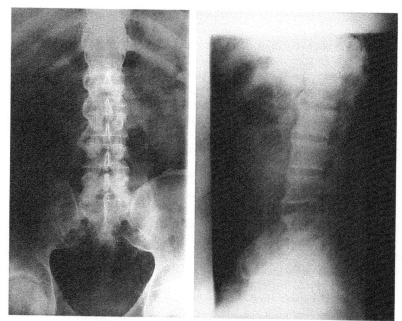

Fig. 1. Bridging osteophytes in idiopathic hypoparathyroidism mimicking diffuse skeletal hyperostosis. (*From* Unverdi S, Oztürk MA, Inal S, et al. Idiopathic hypoparathyroidism mimicking diffuse idiopathic skeletal hyperostosis. J Clin Rheumatol 2009;15:361–2; with permission.)

Systemic Lupus Erythematosus and Rheumatoid Arthritis

Systemic lupus erythematosus (SLE) is known to potentially affect any organ system, and hypoparathyroidism has been found to occur in 4.0% to 5.7% of patients with SLE compared with 1.0% in the general population.[11,12] Hypoparathyroidism is often diagnosed first or simultaneously but one recent case had SLE diagnosed after known hypoparathyroidism.[13] Attout and colleagues[14] and Nashi and colleagues[15] reported cases of hypoparathyroidism detected incidentally in subjects suffering from SLE. They proposed that hypoparathyroidism is underestimated because it is poorly manifested clinically. Hypocalcemia can be precipitated by certain aggravating factors, such as corticosteroid treatment or vitamin D deficiency.

Although acute hypocalcemia typically gives symptoms and signs of musculoskeletal irritability, chronic hypocalcemia usually gives mild symptoms and can even be asymptomatic. Despite the possible lack of outward manifestations, hypocalcemia may be a significant health risk due to prolongation of the QT interval and the consequent risk of sudden death. These cases raise the question of whether periodic calcium and phosphate screening should be routine care for patients with SLE.[15]

For some time, autoimmunity has been implicated in the pathogenesis of hypoparathyroidism and in a subset of patients with this disease antiparathyroid antibodies can be demonstrated.[16–18] A mechanistic link has been drawn between these antibodies and hypoparathyroidism by the demonstration that some antiparathyroid antibodies are able to interfere with secretion of parathyroid hormone and some are directly cytotoxic to bovine parathyroid tissue.[17,18] However, not all antiparathyroid antibodies have a demonstrable physiologic effect.[18] Recently, antibodies against the parathyroid calcium-sensing receptor were found to be significantly more prevalent in subjects with hypoparathyroidism than in normal controls: 49.0% versus 13.3%.[19]

The association between hypoparathyroidism and rheumatoid arthritis (RA) is rare. Edmons and colleagues[20] reported the case of a female subject with longstanding RA and Sjogren syndrome who had a subclinical hypocalcemia. Salvador and colleagues[21] also reported a case. The latter subject, with a previous history of isolated primary hypoparathyroidism, after several years of follow-up, developed a clinical picture suggestive of palindromic rheumatism and, subsequently, a seropositive erosive RA. There is recent evidence of a generalized T-cell activation of peripheral lymphocytes in patients with hypoparathyroidism.[22]

Neuromyotonia, Myopathy, and Rhabdomyolysis

Hypocalcemia caused by hypoparathyroidism has been associated with neuromyotonia (NMT), myopathy, and rhabdomyolysis. Zambelis and colleagues[23] presented a patient with hypoparathyroidism with clinical and electrophysiological findings of neuromyotonia. The patient had the typical clinical findings of hypoparathyroidism. On the other hand, the patient also showed clinical findings typical of NMT: stiffness, paresthesias, and delayed relaxation following voluntary muscle contraction (pseudomyotonia) without visible myokymia. The myokymia and NMT are caused by hyperexcitability of motor nerves and hypocalcemia provokes spontaneous motor unit discharges by lowering the excitability threshold of peripheral nerve axons.[24]

Myopathy is well recognized in hypocalcemia associated with osteomalacia, but the serum creatine kinase (CK) is normal. The association between hypocalcemia and a raised serum CK concentration has been reported in hypoparathyroidism but is not widely recognized.[25] In some reports, the CK level varies inversely with the serum calcium concentration. The combination of rash and raised CK can raise the possibility of dermatomyositis, but this can be excluded by biopsy and resolution of these features with treatment of the hypocalcemia. Barber and colleagues[25] illustrated the importance of checking the serum calcium in patients with muscular symptoms and the clinical value of effective treatment of hypocalcemia.

Hypocalcemia caused by hypoparathyroidism or nonparathyroid disease may, as noted above, be associated with elevated serum levels of the muscle enzymes, and in some patients the enzyme activity may be markedly increased. Akmal[26] reported a case of rhabdomyolysis associated with hypocalcemia caused by idiopathic hypoparathyroidism. The mechanisms of the elevated muscle enzyme activity in patients with hypocalcemia are not well understood. Regardless of the mechanisms, the elevated serum muscle enzymes in patients with hypocalcemia particularly caused by hypoparathyroidism should be recognized and treated appropriately.

Miscellaneous

Subcutaneous calcifications may be seen in the course of hypoparathyroidism, especially about the hips and shoulders.[27] The deposits are generally asymptomatic, although painful calcific periarthritis is reported in this condition, perhaps caused by depression of serum calcium levels.[28] Primary hypoparathyroidism with adhesive capsulitis of the shoulder in the same subject was reported by Harzy and colleagues[29] in a father and daughter. Other patients with hypoparathyroidism have had calcific periarthritis and enthesopathy[30]

Calcification of the basal ganglia occurs in some patients with hypoparathyroidism and is commonly referred to as Fahr syndrome.[31] Although they may be associated with choreoathetosis or a Parkinsonian syndrome, such calcifications may also be asymptomatic.

Both an acquired demyelinating neuropathy and hypoparathyroidism have been found in 2 subjects with polyneuropathy, organomegaly, endocrinopathy, M protein, and skin (POEMS) syndrome.[32] Autoimmune polyendocrine syndrome type 1(APS-1) often includes hypoparathyroidism along with other endocrine deficiencies that can produce musculoskeletal problems. Specific antibodies against NALP5 are found in about half of patients with APS-1 and hypoparathyroidism.[33]

One subject has been reported with hypoparathyroidism developing in a case of cartilage hair hypoplasia (CHH).[34] CHH is a rare autosomal recessive syndrome with severe multisystemic pathology, with immune deficiency, autoimmunity and growth retardation, hair abnormality, panbronchiolitis, hematological symptoms, malabsorption, and chronic diarrhea. CHH is probably linked to autoantibodies directed against the Ca-SR. The Ca-SR is almost ubiquitously expressed in the human body, mainly in the parathyroid cell and the renal tubular cell. In the parathyroid cell, when serum calcium increases, the Ca-SR is activated and inhibits PTH gene expression. Inhibiting mutations in the Ca-SR gene can induce hypercalcemia and hypocalciuria; whereas, activating mutations induce hypocalcemia and hypercalciuria. Symptomatic activating autoantibodies directed against the Ca-SR can be isolated or associated with other immune pathologies.[35]

Pseudohypoparathyroidism and Pseudo Pseudohypoparathyroidism

Pseudohypoparathyroidism (PHP) was first described in 1942 by Albright with a report of a subject with a stocky build, short stature, round facies, brachydactyly, soft-tissue ossifications, and mental retardation[36] a phenotype subsequently known as Albright Hereditary Osteodystrophy. Albright's subject also had hypocalcemic seizures and resistance to parathyroid hormone, thus the condition was termed *pseudohypoparathyroidism*.[37] Albright's hereditary osteodystrophy comprises a distinctive constellation of developmental and skeletal defects consisting of obesity; short, stocky physique; round face; brachydactyly; subcutaneous ossification; and endocrine dysfunction, such as multiple hormone resistance and mental retardation. In most of the reports regarding pseudo pseudohypoparathyroidism (PPHP), metacarpal shortening is observed in the first, fourth, and fifth digits (**Fig. 2**); metatarsal shortening shows predilection for the first and fourth digits.[38] Shortening of the distal phalanx of the thumb is also common. Similar brachydactyly without hypocalcemia has been described as PPHP. This specific pattern of shortening of the bones in the hand may be useful in distinguishing PPHP from other unrelated syndromes in which brachydactyly occurs, such as familial brachydactyly, Turner syndrome, and Klinefelter syndrome.[39]

HYPERPARATHYROIDISM

Hyperparathyroidism (HPT) is caused by increased activity of the parathyroid glands.[40] Primary HPT is a disease originated by hypersecretion of the parathyroid hormone. It is the main cause of hypercalcemia, with an annual rate of 1 case for each 500 women and 2000 men. Asymptomatic disease is common and severe disease with renal stones and metabolic bone disease arises less frequently now than it did 20 to 30 years ago. Secondary HPT is the response of the parathyroid to hypocalcemia of some cause, such as chronic renal failure, osteomalacia, rickets, and malabsorption. Tertiary HPT is a state of autonomous secretion of parathyroid hormone regardless of serum calcium and generally occurs after longstanding secondary HPT. The most common cause of tertiary HPT is end stage chronic kidney

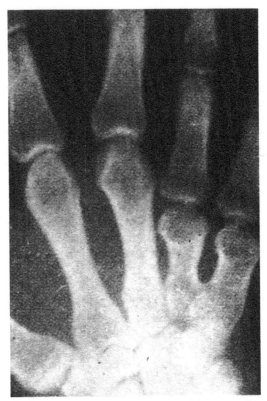

Fig. 2. Short fourth and fifth metacarpal bones in pseudohypoparathyroidism.

disease.[40] Excess parathyroid hormone produced by these diseases can cause many musculoskeletal manifestations.[41–43]

Osteitis Fibrosa Cystic

Osteitis fibrosa cystic (OFC) is the result of extensive bone marrow fibrosis and increased osteoclastic bone reabsorption. Bone resorption occurs because of increased osteoclastic activity and affects all bone surfaces at different skeletal sites. It may be subperiosteal, intracortical, endosteal, trabecular, subchondral, subligamentous, or subtendinous.[44]

A brown tumor is a form of fibrous cystic osteitis, which represents the terminal stage of the bone remodeling process during primary or secondary hyperparathyroidism. Increased PTH levels and locally produced tumor necrosis factor and interleukin (IL)-1 by marrow monocytes induce the proliferation and differentiation of pluripotent bone marrow cells into osteoblasts. These cells produce granulocyte macrophage colony stimulating factor, IL-6, IL-11, and stem-cell factor that induce the migration and differentiation of monocytes into osteoclasts, increasing the number of the latter in the bone tissue. Enhanced activity of osteoclasts and osteoblasts leads to bone resorption and a reduction of bone mineral concentration with an increased proliferation of fibrous tissue and extracellular matrix.[45] Brown tumors develop in 3% to 4% of patients with primary hyperparathyroidism and in 1.5% to 1.7% of patients with secondary causes of hyperparathyroidism[46] Up to half of patients with chronic kidney failure may develop OFC caused by secondary hyperparathyroidism making brown tumors more frequent in these patients. Brown tumors are either monostotic or polyostotic benign masses, painless, and usually found incidentally. However, they may cause tissue damage to adjacent structures and compressive manifestations, such as pain, neuropathies,[47] and myelopathy.[48] The majority of cases report the maxilla and mandible as the main sites of occurrence.[49] Other common sites are the clavicles, scapula, pelvis, and ribs; however, these lesions may appear in any osseous structure,[50] including chondral tissue.[51] They are associated with an increased risk of fractures if localized in weight-bearing areas.[52] Histologically, brown tumors are composed of spindle-shaped mononuclear elements mixed with a certain number of multinuclear giant cells resembling osteoclastic cells and hemorrhagic infiltrates, which gives the tumor a brownish color.[53] Actually they represent a reparative cellular process rather than a true neoplasia. These tumors are usually soft, painless, minimally tender, appear elastic on palpation, and need no specific treatment in most cases. When brown tumors affect the face, they can cause disfiguring deformities and difficulties to breathe through the nose or to eat.[54,55]

On radiograph imaging, brown tumors appear as lytic lesions with thinned cortical bone that may be fractured. Concurrent changes that suggest OFC, such as osteopenia, a salt-and-pepper bone appearance, subperiosteal bone resorption, and disappearance of the lamina dura around the roots of the teeth may help differentiate them from other entities.[56] Tomographic imaging shows an osseous mass, with no cortical disruption, no periosteal reaction or inflammatory signs, a heterogeneous center, and areas that suggest cysts.[52] MRI shows variable intensities on T2-weighted images and intense enhancement on T1-weighted contrast MRI. MRI may be better for determining the presence of cysts or fluid-filled levels, a finding that is suggestive of a brown tumor.[52]

Subperiosteal or Articular Erosions

Subperiosteal bone resorption is the most characteristic radiographic feature of hyperparathyroidism and is found in the phalanges, humerus, and distal epiphysis of the clavicles.[56–58] When resorption is subchondral, such as in the sacroiliac joints, sternoclavicular and acromioclavicular, or the pubic symphysis, it can produce pseudowidening of the joint.[44] Intracortical and endosteal resorption can cause scalloped defects of the inner cortical contour. Subligamentous and subtendinous bone resorption also occurs at many sites, such as the ischial tuberosities, femoral trochanters, and insertions of the coracoclavicular ligaments.[44] Losses of lamina dura of the teeth are also usually caused by bone resorption.

Radiograph evidence of subperiosteal bone resorption (saw-tooth erosions), typical of hyperparathyroidism, is most often seen along the shafts of the phalanges (**Fig. 3**), but when near the joints may resemble the erosions of rheumatoid arthritis. Bywaters has shown some cases in which joint lesions seemed to be caused by collapse or resorption of subchondral and juxta-articular bone.[59] Chondrocalcinosis may also have been a factor in some of these. Erosive arthritis at the hands and wrists has also been seen. In a cross-sectional single-center study of 73 subjects with chronic hemodialysis with hyperparathyroidism, the most common abnormality was subperiosteal bone resorption, mostly at the phalanges and distal clavicles (94% of subjects).[60]

Deformities and Fragility Fractures

In severe cases of hyperparathyroidism, some bone deformities and fragility fractures may appear. Excessive resorption of the terminal phalanges may cause acroosteolysis that may only be detected on hand radiographs.[44] Deformities can cause bone

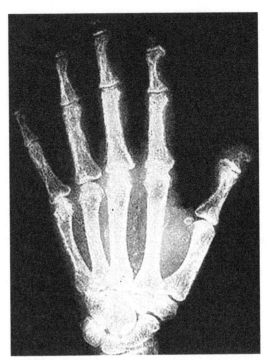

Fig. 3. Radiograph of hyperparathyroidism showing subperiosteal reabsorption, especially along distal second phalanx.

pain, respiratory disorders, and walking disabilities. Severe resorption in the sacroiliac joint may cause great damage to the pelvis, thus leading to deformities that can impair the ability to walk. Thoracic vertebral fractures increase the anteroposterior diameter and enlarge the base, and thus the thorax can take on a bell-mouth shape. In cases of thoracic kyphoscoliosis, abnormal curvature and vertebral rotation may lead to chest deformity.

Fragility fractures sometimes occur at the sites of brown tumors. Because brown tumors are usually painless, the clinical diagnosis is commonly made when patients present with a fracture. In a group of severe secondary hyperparathyroidism, pathologic fractures and deformities were seen in 27% and 33%, respectively. Souza and colleagues[61] have reported a 72-year-old woman with delayed diagnosis of primary hyperparathyroidism, produced by an intrathoracic adenoma, with a longstanding course, presenting with severe osteoporosis, multiple fractures, bone deformities, brown tumor, and neurologic impairments.

Chondrocalcinosis, Calcium Pyrophosphate Crystal Deposition, and Pseudogout

Chondrocalcinosis has been seen in 18% to 25% of patients with hyperparathyroidism.[62,63] Up to 7.5% of patients presenting with what appears to be chondrocalcinosis may be proved to have hyperparathyroidism.[41]

Calcium pyrophosphate crystal deposition (CPPD) disease is diagnosed when CPPD crystals are identified in joint fluid. Their presence is often associated with typical radiographic findings, including fibrocartilage (chondrocalcinosis) or joint capsule calcification. Frequently affected sites include the menisci of the knee, the symphysis pubis, the triangular discs of the distal radioulnar joint, and the glenoid and acetabular labra. Most patients with CPPD disease are asymptomatic, but acute crystal synovitis or chronic arthropathy can be present.[43,64]

An association between hyperparathyroidism and CPPD has been observed in numerous case series.[65–68] All of these studies found that older age increased the risk for radiographic evidence of CPPD. This association could be a result of longer exposure to elevated serum calcium levels, or of age-related changes in cartilage, which might make it more vulnerable to calcification. The proteoglycans that normally inhibit calcium pyrophosphate crystallization[69] might be overwhelmed by the abnormally increased serum calcium levels.[66,67]

Acute pseudogout is a complication of CPPD disease. It involves an acute attack of CPPD crystal-induced synovitis and clinically resembles gout, although the knee, metacarpophalangeal joints, and wrists (not the first metatarsophalangeal joint) are more often affected. Pseudogout has been observed in patients with hyperparathyroidism,[70] especially in the setting of normalization of serum calcium after parathyroid surgery,[71–74] although this association has been questioned.[65,66]

Wang and colleagues[75] described 6 subjects who had primary hyperparathyroidism and pseudogout, 3 of whom developed pseudogout at the nadir of serum calcium after curative parathyroidectomy. In a similar report, Bilezikian and colleagues[71] reported 4 cases of acute arthritis that occurred within 10 days of parathyroidectomy for hyperparathyroidism. All the cases had radiographic findings of CPPD; 2 had intracellular rhomboidal crystals with weakly positive birefringence in joint fluid. In 1989, 20 subjects with primary hyperparathyroidism and pseudogout were described.[76] Eight participants had been diagnosed previously with CPPD; whereas, the others were diagnosed after parathyroidectomy. In another report, an attempt to prevent postoperative pseudogout was described in 3 hyperparathyroid subjects with radiographic CPPD, who received immediate, aggressive vitamin D treatment.[77]

A pseudogout attack after parathyroid surgery appears to be triggered by a decrease in serum calcium, which presumably causes a decrease in calcium concentration in the synovial fluid, making the CPPD crystals more soluble so that they are released from their tissue deposits[78] and shed into the synovial space.[79] Pseudogout attacks have been reported when medical treatment precipitates hypocalcemia. One report described a case of pseudogout in the setting of mithramycin treatment for hypercalcemia,[80] and another in the setting of hypocalcemia after pamidronate treatment.[81]

Gout

Gout, or monosodium urate (MSU) crystal deposition disease, is characterized by attacks of acute inflammatory arthritis in the setting of extracellular urate supersaturation. The incidence of gout appears to be increased in patients with primary hyperparathyroidism.[43,82,83] Thus, CPPD and urate crystals may appear together in joint fluid (**Fig. 4**). In one report, a lytic lesion initially assumed to be a brown tumor was found on joint aspiration to contain urate deposits.[83] A possible explanation for the association of gout and hyperparathyroidism is the increased levels of serum urate that have been described in some,[84] but not all,[85] cohorts of subjects with primary hyperparathyroidism. In one study that described subjects with more severe primary hyperparathyroidism than is commonly seen in the United States, 53 subjects were compared with age-matched and sex-matched controls. The subjects with hyperparathyroidism had significantly higher serum urate levels and reduced clearance of urate.[84] A distinction between diminished excretion or enhanced reabsorption of urate was not made. Serum urate levels were later compared in 26 of the subjects who underwent parathyroidectomy; a significant decrease in serum urate levels was found

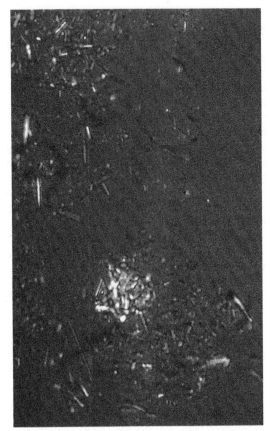

Fig. 4. Monosodium urate and CPPD in joint fluid in hyperparathyroidism.

within 6 months. However, urate levels did not correlate with levels of serum calcium, PTH, or markers of bone turnover.[84]

Myopathy, Proximal Neuromyopathy

Myopathy resembling polymyositis has been described.[86] Some cases of myopathy in secondary hyperparathyroidism have been caused by ischemia. In secondary HPT in chronic renal failure, arterial calcifications with ischemic myopathy and skin ulcers have been reported and create confusion with classic connective tissue disease.[60,87] Myopathy, in at least some primary hyperparathyroidism, has a neurogenic basis.[88] Neuromuscular manifestations of primary hyperparathyroidism typically present as proximal weakness with atrophy and brisk deep tendon reflexes. Hyperparathyroidism has also been possibly implicated in an amyotrophic lateral sclerosis (ALS)-like syndrome with bulbar weakness, fasciculations, and long-tract signs.[89] The pathogenesis of primary hyperparathyroid myopathies is thought to result from a combination of PTH-induced muscle breakdown and altered muscle energy metabolism and use.[89–92] CK levels are normal or slightly elevated. Electromyographic features may be neurogenic or myopathic.[93] Muscle biopsies demonstrate nonspecific features.[94] Typically, if caused by hyperparathyroidism, symptoms will resolve several weeks after parathyroidectomy.[95] Molina reported a subject with myotonic dystrophy and associated primary hyperthyroidism and hyperparathyroidism. At surgery, a parathyroid adenoma was extirpated, and a subtotal thyroidectomy was performed. After surgery, the subject reported subjective improvement in muscle strength.[96] Rymanowski reported an 84-year-old woman with dropped head syndrome caused by primary hyperparathyroidism.[97]

Tendon Ruptures and Avulsions

Parathyroid hormone has been reported to increase bone collagenase and accelerate degradation of insoluble collagen. This finding may be a factor in the occasionally described joint laxity, which, when resulting in hypermobility, could contribute to arthropathy. Tendon rupture and avulsions may be caused by a similar mechanism or to bone resorption as discussed previously at the site of tendon insertions (**Fig. 5**). In 1972, Preston first reported hyperparathyroidism in patients who had avulsion of both quadriceps tendons.[98] From then on, tendon ruptures associated with severe secondary hyperparathyroidism have been reported.[99]

Tendon ruptures occur mostly in weight-bearing tendons. The quadriceps, Achilles tendon, and patellar tendons are most frequently affected. In the upper extremity, the triceps brachii is most commonly involved.[100] Bilateral and unilateral ruptures of the triceps tendon have been reported. Radiological evidence of secondary hyperparathyroidism has been reported as present in 74% of dialysis cases with tendon rupture.[101] Parathyroid hormone has been shown to increase bone resorption at the periosteum and bone marrow interface, suggesting increased osteoclastic activity.[102] A retrospective analysis of subjects on dialysis with a tendon rupture demonstrated marked bone erosions at the site of tendon insertion before tendon injury.[103] Histologic examination of the ruptured tendons from 3 subjects with secondary hyperparathyroidism showed minute bone fragments adjacent to the tendon. The bone demonstrated resorptive lacunae with osteoclasts present on the surface of the

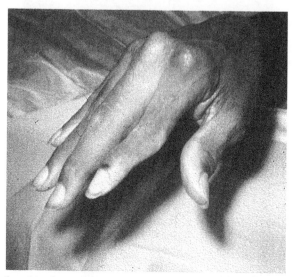

Fig. 5. Finger deformities from subperiosteal erosion and tendon avulsions in a patient with hyperparathyroidism.

trabeculae of the bone fragments.[104] It is likely that secondary hyperparathyroidism leads to osteoclastic bone resorption at the tendon insertion, resulting in multiple avulsion fractures, and contributing to eventual rupture. In one recent study of 65 cases of spontaneous quadriceps tendon rupture, 37% were associated with stage 5 CKD; most affected subjects also had secondary hyperparathyroidism. On examination, patients with quadriceps tendon rupture are unable to extend their knees, may have a knee joint effusion, and have a low-lying patella with a suprapatellar gap. Tendon rupture onset is usually sudden and often occurs without antecedent trauma or extreme exercise. Frequent symptoms include severe pain, stiffness, and difficulty with movement. Physical examination may reveal swelling, warmth, erythema, palpable tenderness, or tendon defects, painful nodules, and subcutaneous bleeding. Ultrasonography or MRI can confirm the diagnosis. The most common site of tendon pathology is the Achilles tendon, but other sites (eg, epicondyle, rotator cuff, finger, or thumb) may be involved.[105] In approximately half of patients, Achilles tendonitis is bilateral.[106]

Rugger-Jersey Spine

At radiography, sclerotic bands along the superior and inferior thoracic and lumbar vertebral body endplates give a striped appearance to the vertebral bodies, with a relative band of lucency at the center of each vertebral body (**Fig. 6**). The alternating

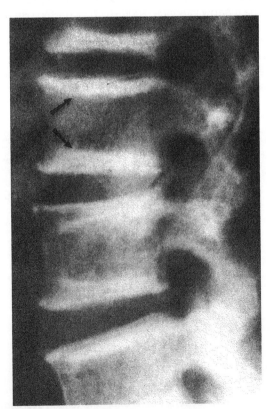

Fig. 6. Radiograph showing rugger-jersey spine in hyperparathyroidism.

parallel sclerotic and lucent bands are analogous to the stripes on an English rugby sweater, from which arises the name *rugger-jersey spine*.[107] The rugger-jersey spine sign is said to be almost diagnostic of the osteosclerosis associated with secondary hyperparathyroidism of chronic renal failure.[108] A rugger-jersey appearance of the spine may result from the demineralization of hyperparathyroidism related either to excessive osteoblastic cell function in response to bone resorption or to increased production of mineralized osteoid. Recently, in a cross-sectional, one-center study, of 73 subjects with chronic hemodialysis and severe hyperparathyroidism, rugger-jersey spine sign was found in 27%.[60]

SUMMARY

Patients with parathyroid disease can have important musculoskeletal problems. Hypoparathyroidism can cause subcutaneous calcifications, tetany, muscle cramps, and paresthesias, but also myopathies and an ankylosing spondylitis-like back disease. Hypoparathyroidism can occur in SLE caused by antiparathyroid antibodies. Patients with hyperparathyroidism can develop bone disease with cysts, erosions, and deformities. They can also develop pseudogout, gout, myopathies, and tendon ruptures.

REFERENCES

1. Shoback D. Hypoparathyroidism. N Engl J Med 2008;359:391–403.
2. Adams JE, Davies M. Paravertebral and peripheral ligamentous ossification: an unusual association of hypoparathyroidism. Postgrad Med J 1977;53:167–72.
3. Goswami R, Ray D, Sharma R, et al. Presence of spondyloarthropathy and its clinical profile in patients with hypoparathyroidism. Clin Endocrinol (Oxf) 2008; 68(2):258–63.
4. Ibn Y, Rostom S, Hajjaj-Hassouni N. Uncommon case of ankylosing spondylitis associated with spontaneous occurring hypoparathyroidism. Rheumatol Int 2009;10:24.
5. Laway BA, Goswami R, Singh N, et al. Pattern of bone mineral density in patients with sporadic idiopathic hypoparathyroidism. Clin Endocrinol 2006; 64:405–9.
6. Sivrioglu K, Ozcakir S, Kamay O. Hypoparathyroidism: a rare cause of spondy-loarthropathy. Scand J Rheumatol 2006;35:494–5.
7. Resnick D, Niwayama G. Radiographic and pathologic features of spinal involvement in diffuse skeletal hyperostosis in idiopathic hypoparathyroidism (DISH). Radiology 1976;119:559–68.
8. Korkmaz C, Yasar S, Binboga A. Hypoparathyroidism simulating ankylosing spondylitis. Joint Bone Spine 2005;72:89–91.
9. Takuwa Y, Matsumoto T, Kurokawa T, et al. Calcium metabolism in paravertebral ligamentous ossification. Acta Endocrinol (Copenh) 1985;109:428–32.
10. Okazaki T, Takuwa Y, Yamamoto M, et al. Ossification of the paravertebral ligaments: a frequent complication of hypoparathyroidism. Metabolism 1984;33: 710–3.
11. McDonagh JE, Isenberg DA. Development of additional autoimmune diseases in a population of patients with systemic lupus erythematosus. Ann Rheum Dis 2000;59:230–2.
12. Pyne D, Isenberg DA. Autoimmune thyroid disease in systemic lupus erythematosus. Ann Rheum Dis 2002;61:70–2.

13. Sahebari M, Afkhamizadeh M, Hashemzadeh K, et al. Development of systemic lupus erythematosus in a patient with hypoparathyroidism: a case report and review of the literature. Int J Rheum Dis 2010;13:175–9.

14. Attout H, Guez S, Durand J, et al. Hypoparathyroidism in systemic lupus erythematosus. Joint Bone Spine 2007;74:282–4.

15. Nashi E, Banerjee D, Crelinsten G. Hypoparathyroidism in systemic lupus erythematosus. Lupus 2005;14:164–5.

16. Posillico JT, Wortsman J, Srikanta S, et al. Parathyroid cell surface autoantibodies that inhibit parathyroid hormone secretion from dispersed human parathyroid cells. J Bone Miner Res 1986;1:475–83.

17. Brandi M-L, Aurbach GD, Fattorossi A, et al. Antibodies cytotoxic to bovine parathyroid cells in autoimmune hypoparathyroidism. Proc Natl Acad Sci U S A 1986;83:8366–9.

18. Li Y, Song YH, Rais N, et al. Autoantibodies to the extracellular domain of the calcium sensing receptor in patients with acquired hypoparathyroidism. J Clin Invest 1996;97:910–4.

19. Goswami R, Brown EM, Kochupillai N, et al. Prevalence of calcium sensing receptor autoantibodies in patients with sporadic idiopathic hypoparathyroidism. Eur J Endocrinol 2004;150:9–18.

20. Edmons ME, Saunders A, Sturrock RD. Rheumatoid arthritis associated with hypoparathyroidism and Sjogren syndrome. J R Soc Med 1979;72:856–8.

21. Salvador G, Sanmarti R, Ros I, et al. Idiopathic hypoparathyroidism associated with adult rheumatoid arthritis. Clin Rheumatol 1999;18:334–6.

22. Wortsman J, McConnachie P, Baker JR, et al. T-lymphocyte activation in adult onset idiopathic hypoparathyroidism. Am J Med 1992;92:352–6.

23. Zambelis T, Licomanos D, Leonardos A, et al. Neuromyotonia in idiopathic hypoparathyroidism. Neurol Sci 2009;30:495–7.

24. Brick FB, Gutmann L, McComas CF. Calcium effect on generation and amplification of myokymic discharges. Neurology 1982;32:618–22.

25. Barber J, Butler RC, Davie M, et al. Hypoparathyroidism presenting as myopathy with raised creatine kinase. Rheumatology 2001;40:1417–8.

26. Akmal M. Rhabdomyolysis in a patient with hypocalcemia due to hypoparathyroidism. Am J Nephrol 1993;13(1):61–3.

27. Steinberg H, Waldron BR. Idiopathic hypoparathyroidism: analysis of 52 cases, including report of new case. Medicine 1952;31:133–8.

28. Walton K, Swinson DR. Acute calcific periarthritis associated with transient hypocalcaemia secondary to hypoparathyroidism. Case report. Br J Rheumatol 1983;22:179–80.

29. Harzy T, Benbouazza K, Amine B, et al. Idiopathic hypoparathyroidism and adhesive capsulitis of the shoulder in two first-degree relatives. Joint Bone Spine 2004;71:234–6.

30. de Carvalho A, Jurik AG, Illum F. Case report 335. Skeletal Radiol 1986;15:52–4.

31. Manyam BV. What is and what is not 'Fahr's disease'. Parkinsonism Relat Disord 2005;11:73–80.

32. Proietti G, Puliti M, Tulli F, et al. A man with worsening weakness. Minerva Med 1999;90:175–7.

33. Alimohammadi M, Björklund P, Haligren A, et al. Autoimmune polyendocrine syndrome type 1 and NALP5, a parathyroid autoantigen. N Engl J Med 2008;358:1018–28.

34. Bacchetta J, Ranchin B, Brunet AS, et al. Autoimmune hypoparathyroidism in a 12-year-old girl with McKusick cartilage hair hypoplasia. Pediatr Nephrol 2009;24:2449–53.
35. Kifor O, McElduff A, LeBoff MS, et al. Activating antibodies to the calcium-sensing receptor in two patients with autoimmune hypoparathyroidism. J Clin Endocrinol Metab 2004;89(2):548–56.
36. Albright F, Burnett CH, Smith PH, et al. Pseudohypoparathyroidism—an example of "Seabright–Bantam syndrome". Endocrinology 1942;30:922–32.
37. Wilson LC, Hall CM. Albright's hereditary osteodystrophy and pseudohypoparathyroidism. Semin Musculoskelet Radiol 2002;6:273–83.
38. Sanctis L, Vai S, Andreo MR, et al. Brachydactyly in 14 genetically characterized pseudohypoparathyroidism type Ia patients. J Clin Endocrinol Metab 2004;89:1650–5.
39. Unlu Z, Orguc S, Ovali GY, et al. Unusual long bone and metacarpo-carpal abnormalities in a case of pseudo-pseudohypoparathyroidism. Clin Rheumatol 2007;26:1155–7.
40. Fraser WD. Hyperparathyroidism. Lancet 2009;374:145–58.
41. Schumacher HR. Arthritis associated with endocrine and metabolic disease. In: Katz WA, editor. Rheumatic disease: diagnosis and management. Philadelphia 1977. p. 682–97.
42. Jacobs-Kosmin D, DeHoratius RJ. Musculoskeletal manifestations of endocrine disorders. Curr Opin Rheumatol 2005;17:64–9.
43. Rubin MR, Silverberg SJ. Rheumatic manifestations of primary hyperparathyroidism and parathyroid hormone therapy. Curr Rheumatol Rep 2002;4:179–85.
44. Jevtic V. Imaging of renal osteodystrophy. Eur J Radiol 2003;46:85–95.
45. Hruska K. New concepts in renal osteodystrophy. Nephrol Dial Transplant 1998;13:2755–60.
46. Takeshita T, Tanaka H, Harasawa A, et al. Brown tumor of the sphenoid sinus in a patient with secondary hyperparathyroidism: CT and MR imaging findings. Radiat Med 2004;22:265–8.
47. Tarrass F, Ayad A, Benjelloun M, et al. Cauda equina compression revealing brown tumor of the spine in a long-term hemodialysis patient. Joint Bone Spine 2006;73:748–50.
48. Kaya RA, Cavusoglu H, Tanik C, et al. Spinal cord compression caused by a brown tumor at the cervicothoracic junction. Spine J 2007;7:728–32.
49. Jeren-Strujic B, Rozman B, Lambasa S, et al. Secondary hyperparathyroidism and brown tumor in dialyzed patients. Ren Fail 2001;23:279–86.
50. Erturk E, Keskin M, Ersoy C, et al. Metacarpal brown tumor in secondary hyperparathyroidism due to vitamin-D deficiency. A case report. J Bone Joint Surg Am 2005;87:1363–6.
51. Perrin J, Zaunbauer W, Haertel M. Brown tumor of the thyroid cartilage: CT findings. Skeletal Radiol 2003;32:530–2.
52. Takeshita T, Takeshita K, Abe S, et al. Brown tumor with fluid-fluid levels in a patient with primary hyperparathyroidism: radiological findings. Radiat Med 2006;24:631–4.
53. Batsakis J. Tumors of the head and neck. Baltimore (MD): Williams &Wilkins; 1979. p. 397–8.
54. Morrone LF, Ettore GC, Passavati G, et al. Maxillary brown tumor in secondary hyperparathyroidism requiring urgent parathyroidectomy. J Nephrol 2001;14:415–9.
55. Tarello F, Ottone S, De Gioanni PP, et al. Brown tumor of the jaws. Minerva Stomatol 1996;45:465–70.

56. Kuhlman JE, Ren H, Hutchins GM, et al. Fulminant pulmonary calcification complicating renal transplantation: CT demonstration. Radiology 1989;173: 459–60.
57. Gavelli G, Zompatori M. Thoracic complications in uremic patients and in patients undergoing dialytic treatment: state of the art. Eur Radiol 1997;7: 708–17.
58. Resnick D, Niwayama G. Subchondral resorption of bone in renal osteodystrophy. Radiology 1976;118:315–21.
59. Grahame R, Sutor DJ, Mitchener MB. Crystal deposition in hyperparathyroidism. Ann Rheum Dis 1971;30:597–604.
60. Lacativa PH, Rranco FM, Pimentel JR, et al. Prevalence of radiological findings among cases of severe secondary hyperparathyroidism. Sao Paulo Med J 2009; 127:71–7.
61. Souza ER, Scrignoli JA, Bezerra FC, et al. Devastating skeletal effects of delayed diagnosis of complicated primary hyperparathyroidism because of ectopic adenoma. J Clin Rheumatol 2008;14:281–4.
62. Dodds WJ, Steinbach HL. Primary hyperparathyroidism and articular cartilage calcification. Am J Roentgenol Radium Ther Nucl Med 1968;104: 884–92.
63. Ryckewaert A, Solnica J, Lanham C, et al. The articular manifestations of hyperparathyroidism. J Belge Rhumatol Med Phys 1966;21:289–302.
64. Doherty M, Dieppe P. Clinical aspects of calcium pyrophosphate dihydrate crystal deposition. Rheum Dis Clin North Am 1988;14:395–414.
65. Huaux JP, Geubel A, Koch MC, et al. The arthritis of hemochromatosis: a review of 25 cases with special reference to chondrocalcinosis and a comparison with patients with primary hyperparathyroidism and controls. Clin Rheumatol 1986;5: 317–24.
66. Pritchard MH, Jessop JD. Chondrocalcinosis in primary hyperparathyroidism: influence of age, metabolic bone disease, and parathyroidectomy. Ann Rheum Dis 1977;36:146–51.
67. McGill PE, Grange AT, Royston CS. Chondrocalcinosis in primary hyperparathyroidism: influence of parathyroid activity and age. Scand J Rheumatol 1984;13: 56–8.
68. Yashiro T, Okamoto T, Tanaka R, et al. Prevalence of chondrocalcinosis in patients with primary hyperparathyroidism in Japan. Endocrinol Jpn 1991; 38(5):457–64.
69. Rynes RI, Merzig EG. Calcium pyrophosphate crystal deposition disease and hyperparathyroidism: a controlled, prospective study. J Rheumatol 1978;5: 460–8.
70. McCarty DJ. Pseudogout: articular chondrocalcinosis: calcium pyrophosphate crystal deposition disease. In: Hollander JL, editor. Arthritis and allied conditions. Philadelphia: Lea & Febiger; 1966. p. 947–64.
71. Bilezikian JP, Connor TB, Aptekar R, et al. Pseudogout after parathyroidectomy. Lancet 1973;1:445–6.
72. Sharp WV, Kelly TR. Acute arthritis: a complication of surgically induced hypoparathyroidism. Am J Surg 1967;113:829–32.
73. O'Duffy JD. Clinical studies of acute pseudogout attacks: comments on prevalence, predispositions, and treatment. Arthritis Rheum 1976;19:349–52.
74. Kobayashi S, Sugenoya A, Takahashi S, et al. Two cases of acute pseudogout attack following parathyroidectomy. Endocrinol Jpn 1991;38:309–14.

75. Wang CA, Miller LM, Weber AL, et al. Pseudogout: a diagnostic clue to hyperparathyroidism. Am J Surg 1969;117:558–65.
76. Geelhoed GW, Kelly TR. Pseudogout as a clue and complication in primary hyperparathyroidism. Surgery 1989;106:1036–41.
77. Yashiro T, Hara H, Ito K, et al. Pseudogout associated with primary hyperparathyroidism: management in the immediate postoperative period for prevention of acute pseudogout attack. Endocrinol Jpn 1988;35:617–24.
78. Bennett RM, Lehr JR, McCarty DJ. Factors affecting the solubility of calcium pyrophosphate dihydrate crystals. J Clin Invest 1975;56:1571–9.
79. McCarty DJ. Calcium pyrophosphate dihydrate crystal deposition disease—1975. Arthritis Rheum 1976;19:275–85.
80. Pieters GF, Mol MJ, Boerbooms AM, et al. Pseudogout attacks after successful treatment of hyperparathyroidism. Neth J Med 1989;34:258–63.
81. Malnick SD, Ariel-Ronen S, Evron E, et al. Acute pseudogout as a complication of pamidronate. Ann Pharmacother 1997;31:499–500.
82. Terkeltaub RA. Pathogenesis and treatment of crystal-induced inflammation. In: Koopman WJ, editor. Arthritis and allied conditions: a textbook of rheumatology. 13th edition. Baltimore (MD): Williams & Wilkins; 1997. p. 2085.
83. Mallette LE, Bilezikian JP, Heath DA, et al. Primary hyperparathyroidism: clinical and biochemical features. Medicine (Baltimore) 1974;53:127–46.
84. Broulik PD, Stepan JJ, Pacovsky V. Primary hyperparathyroidism and hyperuricaemia are associated but not correlated with indicators of bone turnover. Clin Chim Acta 1987;170:195–200.
85. Silverberg SJ, Shane E, Jacobs TP, et al. A 10-year prospective study of primary hyperparathyroidism with or without parathyroid surgery. N Engl J Med 1999;341:1249–55.
86. Frame B, Heinze EG Jr, Block MA, et al. Myopathy in primary hyperparathyroidism. Observations in three patients. Ann Intern Med 1968;68:1022–7.
87. Coen G, Mantella D, Sardella D, et al. Asymmetric dimethylarginine, vascular calcifications and parathyroid hormone serum levels in hemodialysis patients. J Nephrol 2009;22:616–22.
88. Patten BM, Bilezikian JP, Mallette LE, et al. Neuromuscular disease in primary hyperparathyroidism. Ann Intern Med 1974;80:182–93.
89. Jackson CE, Amato AA, Bryan WW, et al. Primary hyperparathyroidism and ALS: is there a relation? Neurology 1998;50:1795–9.
90. Baczynski R, Massry SG, Magott M, et al. Effect of parathyroid hormone on energy metabolism of skeletal muscle. Kidney Int 1985;28:722–7.
91. Garber AJ. Effects of parathyroid hormone on skeletal muscle protein and amino acid metabolism in the rat. J Clin Invest 1983;71:1806–21.
92. Smogorzewski M, Piskorska G, Borum PR, et al. Chronic renal failure, parathyroid hormone and fatty acids oxidation in skeletal muscle. Kidney Int 1988;33:555–60.
93. Kendall-Taylor P, Turnbull DM. Endocrine myopathies. Br Med J (Clin Res Ed) 1983;287:705–8.
94. Ruff RL, Weissmann J. Endocrine myopathies. Neurol Clin 1988;6:575–92.
95. Beekman R, Tijssen CC, Visser LH, et al. Dropped head as the presenting symptom of primary hyperparathyroidism. J Neurol 2002;249:1738–9.
96. Molina MJ, Lara JI, Riobo P. Primary hyperthyroidism and associated hyperparathyroidism in a patient with myotonic dystrophy: Steinert with hyperthyroidism and hyperparathyroidism. Am J Med Sci 1996;311:296–8.

97. Rymanowski JV, Twydell PT. Treatable dropped head syndrome in hyperparathyroidism. Muscle Nerve 2009;39:409–10.

98. Preston ET. Avulsion of both quadriceps tendons in hyperparathyroidism. JAMA 1972;221:406–7.

99. Palmer S, Birks C, Dunbar J, et al. Simultaneous multiple tendon ruptures complicating a seizure in a haemodialysis patient. Nephrology (Carlton) 2004; 9:262–4.

100. Tsourvakas S, Gouvalas K, Gimtsas C, et al. Bilateral and simultaneous rupture of the triceps tendons in chronic renal failure and secondary hyperparathyroidism. Arch Orthop Trauma Surg 2004;124:278–80.

101. Jones N, Kjellstrand C. Spontaneous tendon ruptures in patients on chronic dialysis. Am J Kidney Dis 1996;28:861–6.

102. Petersen J, Kang B. In vivo effect of b2-microglobulin on bone resorption. Am J Kidney Dis 1994;23:726–30.

103. Meneghello A, Bertoli M. Tendon disease and adjacent bone erosions in dialysis patients. Br J Radiol 1983;56:915–20.

104. Ryuzaki M, Konishi K, Kasuga A, et al. Spontaneous rupture of the quadriceps tendon in patients on maintenance haemodialysis: report of three cases with clinicopathological observations. Clin Nephrol 1989;32:144–8.

105. Shah MK. Simultaneous bilateral quadriceps tendon rupture in renal patients. Clin Nephrol 2002;58:118–21.

106. Muzi F, Gravante G, Tati E, et al. Fluoroquinolones-induced tendinitis and tendon rupture in kidney transplant recipients: 2 cases and a review of the literature. Transplant Proc 2007;39:1673–5.

107. Karani S. Secondary hyperparathyroidism: primary renal failure. Proc R Soc Med 1955;48:527–30.

108. Wittenberg A. The rugger jersey spine sign. Radiology 2004;230:491–2.

Osteoporosis and Osteomalacia

Linda A. Russell, MD

KEYWORDS

• Osteoporosis • Osteomalacia • Vitamin D deficiency
• Chronic kidney disease

Metabolic bone disease is becoming a more recognized disease entity. Endocrine disease often is associated with metabolic bone disease. This article attempts to delineate the current knowledge of osteoporosis and osteomalacia in endocrine diseases. The World Health Organization (WHO) defines osteopenia as when the dual energy x-ray absorptiometry (DEXA) T-score in a postmenopausal women is between −1.0 and −2.4, and osteoporosis as when the T-score is −2.5 or lower. The bone is normal, but there is an increased risk of fracture because of fragility of the bone. Osteomalacia refers to bone that is abnormal because of abnormal mineralization. The most common cause of osteomalacia is vitamin D deficiency.

HYPERTHYROIDISM

Thyroid hormones have a direct resorptive effect on bone. Low thyroid-stimulating hormone (TSH) and high thyroxine (T_4) levels can exert a negative effect on bone resorption.[1] Hyperthyroid patients have a significant negative calcium balance. Bone loss occurs more in cortical than trabecular bone. Hyperthyroid states can be compartmentalized into overt hyperthyroidism, endogenous subclinical hyperthyroidism, and exogenous subclinical hyperthyroidism due to suppressive therapy and thyroid hormone replacement therapy. Overt hyperthyroidism and iatrogenic hyperthyroidism result in significant osteoporosis and fractures. A recent study[2] demonstrated that bone mineral density and level of bone-turnover markers were significantly more favorable in 115 subjects with TSH level between 0.35 and 6.3mU/L than in women with a TSH level less than 0.3 mU/L. It has been estimated that more than 10% of postmenopausal women in the United States receive thyroid hormone replacement and up to 20% of these women are over-replaced, inducing subclincal hyperthyroidism.[3]

Overt hyperthyroidism requires rapid correction of the thyrotoxicosis to prevent skeletal and other manifestations of this syndrome. Data do suggest that treatment

No Financial Disclosures.

Weill Cornell School of Medicine, Hospital for Special Surgery, 535 East 70th Street, New York, NY 10021, USA

E-mail address: russelll@hss.edu

of endogenous subclinical hyperthyroidism can minimize further loss of bone density.[4] Treatments with estrogen[5] and bisphosphonates[6] seem to prevent thyroid hormone-mediated bone loss.

HYPERPARATHYROIDISM

Hyperparathyroidism is divided into primary and secondary hyperparathyroidism (**Table 1**). Classically, primary hyperparathyroidism is recognized as a disease of "bones, stones, and groans"; now, the condition is asymptomatic in most patients because the current biochemical profile contains serum calcium, and markedly high levels of calcium are detected sooner than in the past. Primary hyperparathyroidism is a generalized disorder of calcium, phosphate, and bone metabolism that results from an increased level of parathyroid hormone (PTH). The prevalence is as high as 1 in 500 to 1 in 1000. Most adults with primary hyperparathyroidism (80%–85%) have a single benign adenoma, whereas 15% to 20% have hyperplasia of all glands.[7] Four-gland hyperplasia is common in patients with chronic kidney disease (CKD) or with multiple endocrine neoplasia Type I or II. Patients with primary hyperthyroidism are at risk of bone loss and osteoporosis. Cortical bone is more affected than trabecular bone; as such, forearm bone mineral density (BMD) is most affected in primary hyperparathyroidism. BMD measurement is essential in all patients with primary hyperparathyroidism. It helps define the extent of disease and helps to monitor ongoing disease activity. A 10-year prospective study of patients with primary hyperparathyroidism who underwent parathyroidectomy demonstrated normalization of biochemical values and increased bone density.[8] The 2002 National Institute of Health guidelines on asymptomatic primary hyperparathyroidism recommend that patients with primary hyperparathyroidism and the following criteria be managed surgically: a calcium level greater than 1.0 mg/dL over the upper limit of normal, a 24-hour urinary calcium excretion level greater than 400 mg, a reduction in creatinine clearance of 30%, a T-score of −2.5 at any site, or age less than 50 years.[7] If these criteria do not apply, patients can be managed nonsurgically. Nonsurgical patients should test serum calcium level every 6 months and BMD of the lumbar spine, hip, and forearm yearly. Patients can maintain a normal amount of calcium and vitamin D.[9] The 2009 International Task Force on the medical management of asymptomatic primary hyperparathyroidism commented that bisphosphonates and hormone replacement therapy reduce bone loss in the population.[10] Calcimimetics are agents that alter the function of the extracellular calcium-sensing receptor and offer an exciting new approach in patients with primary hyperparathyroidism. In these patients, calcimimetics may reduce serum calcium and PTH levels but have no beneficial effect on bone turnover; further study is needed, in this area.[11] Frequently, patients who undergo removal of a parathyroid adenoma require only observation, because BMD often improves rapidly.

Table 1 Hyperparathyroidism		
	Calcium	PTH Level
Primary	↑	↑
Secondary	↓	↑
Secondary	normal	↑
Hypercalcemia Unrelated to PTH	↑	↓

Abbreviation: PTH, parathyroid hormone.

Secondary hyperparathyroidism is common and is due to inadequate calcium and vitamin D intake. It is essential to evaluate patients with osteopenia or osteoporosis for secondary osteoporosis and to correct calcium or vitamin D deficiency. This helps attain maximal response to additional pharmacologic therapy prescribed. It is best to correct significant secondary hyperparathyroidism before initiating antiresorptive or anabolic therapy (**Table 2**).

HYPOPARATHYROIDISM

Hypothyroidism is an uncommon disease caused by insufficient PTH. The most common causes are immunologic destruction, radiation therapy, and surgical removal. Patients develop hypocalcemia and hyperphosphatemia. Idiopathic hypophosphatemia can lead to various musculoskeletal findings, including diffuse ligamentous and entheseal ossifications. A recent report describes a 50-year-old man with idiopathic hypoparathyroidism who was diagnosed with diffuse idiopathic skeletal hyperostosis when 40 years old.[12]

The treatment usually consists of replacement of calcium and calcitriol and being sure to avoid hypercalciuria, which increases the risk of nephrolithiasis. Phosphate binders, such as calcium acetate (PhosLo), sevelamer (Renagel), and lanthanum (Fosrenol), can be used for resistant hyperphosphatemia. Several studies have looked at the use of intact PTH as a treatment for this condition. Patients seem to require less calcium and calcitriol when given PTH.[13] Patients treated with PTH also seem to have correction of the low bone-turnover state associated with hypothyroidism.[14]

VITAMIN D DEFICIENCY

Vitamin D deficiency has received much attention over the past few years with the recognition of the many people deficient in Vitamin D living in northern latitudes. Vitamin D is obtained from cutaneous production when 7-dehydrocholesterol is converted to vitamin D_3 (cholecalciferol) by ultraviolet B radiation or by oral intake of vitamin D_2 (ergocalciferol) or vitamin D_3. Fatty fish is the most important dietary source. Fortification of foods is practiced in some countries, including the United States; however, the standardization of this process is poor. After production in the skin, vitamin D is hydroxylated in the liver to 25-hydroxyvitamin D [25(OH)D], which is further hydroxylated in the kidney to 1, 25(OH)D, the active metabolite. Vitamin D is usually assessed by measuring the serum concentration of 25(OH)D.[15] There is increasing agreement that the optimal circulating level of 25(OH)D should be approximately 30 to 32 ng/mL or greater.[9] Ideally, the optimal vitamin D level maximally

Table 2	
Treatment of secondary hyperparathyroidism	
Replacement of calcium	
Calcium citrate 500 mg 3–4 times per day	
Replacement of vitamin D	
Vitamin D (ng/ml)	
<20	Ergocalciferol (Drisdol) 50,000 IU/wk + vitamin D_3 1000–2000 iu/d
20–30	Vitamin D_3 2000–5000 IU/d
>30	Vitamin D_3 1000–2000 IU/d

25-Hydroxyvitamin D_3 and intact PTH levels can be checked every 6 weeks and dosages adjusted as necessary.

suppresses PTH; this would ensure adequate intake of vitamin D. It is thought that the recommendation for daily vitamin D would eventually be to keep the serum vitamin D level well above the current recommendation of 32 ng/mL.

Epidemiology

Elderly patients have been found to have decreased dermal synthesis. Older nursing home residents frequently do not go outdoors often and are not exposed to sunshine on a regular basis. In a meta-analysis of randomized controlled trials, a dosage of 700 to 800 IU/d of vitamin D was found to reduce the relative risk of hip fracture by 26% and any new vertebral fractures by23% versus calcium or placebo.[16] There have been smaller studies that failed to show the benefit of vitamin D in fracture reduction, but a Cochrane review did show benefit in fracture reduction when both calcium and vitamin D supplements were given.[17] It has been shown that low vitamin D levels are associated with muscle weakness and an increased risk of falls.[5,18]

25(OH)D is the major form of circulating vitamin D, but 1, 25(OD)D (calcitriol) is the active metabolite. This metabolite binds to the nuclear vitamin D receptor (VDR). By binding to the appropriate receptor, vitamin D can stimulate intestinal calcium absorption, stimulate bone resorption, and decrease PTH secretion. Vitamin D seems to be able to enhance receptor-activated nuclear factor-κB ligand (RANKL) and osteoprotegerin (OPG) and stimulate osteoclast formation and genes involved in bone formation, such as osteocalcin and osteopontin[19,20] Vitamin D deficiency results in poor mineralization of the growth plate, which becomes thick, wide, and irregular. In adults who are vitamin D-deficient, the newly formed bone matrix, the osteoid, does not mineralize. Vitamin D receptors exist on many cells other than bone cells and active investigation is under way to investigate other functions of vitamin D.

Clinical Aspects of Vitamin D Deficiency

Rickets presents with decreased longitudinal growth, widening of the epiphyseal zones, and painful swelling around involved joints, with bowing of the tibia caused by poor mineralization and swelling of rib cartilage. Children evidence developmental delay. Osteomalacia can be associated with bone pain, muscle weakness, and difficulty walking. Proximal muscle is affected more than distal strength, so activities such as climbing stairs and getting out of a low chair can be particularly difficult.

Rickets and osteomalacia are often seen when vitamin D levels get to 10 ng/mL or lower.[21] Coexistent laboratory findings often include hypocalcemia, hypophosphatemia, and elevated alkaline phosphate level. PTH levels are usually elevated, suggesting a component of secondary hyperparathyroidism.

Radiographs in patients with rickets reveal decreased mineralization around the epiphysis, unsharp bone margins, and less contrast. These findings rapidly improve with treatment. In osteomalacia, radiographs show less contrast and are less sharp. Looser zones represent pseudofractures. These areas can also be seen on bone scan. DEXA results can improve rapidly with treatment.

Treatment of Vitamin D Deficiency

Rickets and osteomalacia are fairly quickly treated with vitamin D supplementation unless there is a component of malabsorption, as in patients with celiac disease or inflammatory bowel disease or who have undergone gastric bypass. Vitamin D_3 can be supplemented at dosages of 1000 to 2000 IU/d. Alternatively, vitamin D_2 (ergocalciferol) can be given at dosages of 50,000 IU/wk. A calcium supplement should always be added. After treatment of vitamin D deficiency, serum calcium and phosphorus levels should correct quickly. PTH levels may lag behind and take some time to normalize, correcting a state of secondary hyperparathyroidism. Children may require lower doses of vitamin supplementation. Vitamin D levels should be followed to ensure repletion.

Vitamin D intoxication is rare. Signs and symptoms may include those of hypercalcemia, such as thirst, polyuria, and headache. Laboratory testing may reveal hypercalcemia and normal or increased phosphate, increased serum creatinine or blood urea nitrogen, very high 25(OH)D, normal 1, 25(OH)D, and suppressed PTH levels. Patients respond to withdrawal of supplemental calcium and vitamin D. Patients with granulomatous diseases or lymphoproliferative disorders have macrophages containing 1α-hydroxalase, thus permitting conversion of 25(OH)D to 1, 25(OH)D. Supplementing these patients with vitamin D should be handled carefully, because vitamin D intoxication can occur much more easily. Glucocorticoids can decrease the hydroxylation of 25(OH)D to 1, 25(OH)D and help reverse this process in this select group of patients.

HYPOPHOSPHATEMIA

The 3 most common causes of hypophosphatemia are redistribution of phosphorus from extracellular fluid into cells, increased urinary excretion, and decreased intestinal absorption. The clinical manifestations depend on the severity of the condition. Early on, hypophosphatemia can cause increased bone resorption. Impaired bone mineralization causes rickets in children and osteomalacia in adults. X-linked hypophosphatemic rickets is the most common disorder of renal wasting, occurring in about 1 of 25,000 live births. A recent report describes lateral subtrochanteric pseudofractures occurring in adults with osteomalacia from hypophosphatasia and X-linked hypophosphatemia, suggesting that a low bone-turnover state played a role in the fractures.[22] A mutation in the type 2a sodium-phosphate cotransporter has been associated hypophosphatemia, nephrolithiasis, and osteoporosis[23]; this mutation results in abnormal renal phosphate reabsorption.

HYPOMAGNESEMIA

Hypomagnesemia is usually caused by loss of magnesium from the gastrointestinal tract or kidney. Hypocalcemia is a common manifestation of moderate-to-severe magnesium depletion. Both can be associated with neuromuscular hyperexcitability and tetany, as elicited by positive Chvostek and Trousseau signs. Epidemiologic studies suggest that a low magnesium diet may be a risk factor of osteoporosis. Magnesium deficiency in rats can cause a decrease in bone mass and skeletal fragility.[24] Magnesium supplements may be associated with increased bone mass.[18] The physician must screen those at risk of hypomagnesemia with a serum magnesium level.

GONADAL STEROIDS

Estrogen and testosterone play an important role in maintaining skeletal architecture. The estrogen and testosterone decrease with aging has profound effects on the skeleton. At menopause, women undergo rapid trabecular bone loss.[25] The duration of rapid bone loss can begin 1 to 2 years before menopause and continue for up to 5 years after, when there can be a loss of 20% to 30% of trabecular bone and 5% to 10% of cortical bone. About 8 to 10 years after menopause, there is a slower and continuous rate of bone loss in which cortical and trabecular bone loss is similar. Men demonstrate slow, equal loss of cortical and trabecular bone from midlife until death. As men reach a higher peak bone density and do not have the accelerated rate of loss that women have at menopause, bone generally does not fracture in men as frequently as in women.

Changes in bone quantity and structure help account for the varying rates of fractures in women and men with aging. Distal forearm fractures increase markedly in women around the time of menopause and plateau about 15 years after menopause. Vertebral and hip fracture rates increase after menopause; then vertebral fracture rate plateaus but hip fracture rate continues to increase. The incidence of vertebral and hip fractures in men parallel that of women but are delayed by one decade, due to the lack of a manpower. Men do not have a significant increase in wrist fractures with aging.

In women, at menopause, there is an increase in the basic multicellular unit activation frequency,[26] an extension of the resorption period,[26] and a shortening of the formation period.[27] Estrogen has a central role in osteoblastic differentiation and limits apoptosis of osteoblasts and osteocytes.[28,29] Estrogen supplementation can have an anabolic effect on bone.[30] Estrogen suppresses production of RANKL and increases production of OPG, which ultimately decreases osteoclastic production and differentiation.[31] Estrogen can also promote apoptosis of osteoclasts.

In men, with aging, there is an increase in sex hormone binding globulin (SHBG) resulting in less bioavailable testosterone and estrogen. Although testosterone is the major sex steroid in men, many studies demonstrate that male BMD at many sites correlates better with bioavailable estradiol levels than testosterone levels.[32,33] Clinically, it is still useful to check testosterone levels in men with osteoporosis or osteomalacia and consider replacement if levels are low.

During pregnancy, there is increased intestinal absorption of calcium, in part, due to increased 1,25(OH)D levels. Although this has not been studied extensively, there is probably no significant change in BMD during pregnancy. During lactation, because of increased parathyroid hormone-related protein (PTHrP) levels, there is increased bone resorption to provide the calcium needed for breast milk (280–400 mg/d). There is also reduced renal excretion of calcium during lactation. Calcitonin may play a role in limiting bone resorption during lactation. The temporary skeletal loss of calcium during lactation is completely restored after weaning. Overall, pregnancy and lactation seem not to have a significant detrimental effect on the maternal skeleton. Women who are vitamin D-deficient during pregnancy also seem to give birth to children with normal skeletons because of increased maternal calcium absorption.

Medications that lower estrogen levels, such as the aromatase inhibitors, are associated with bone loss and fractures. Depo-Provera suppresses menstruation and is associated with bone loss and fracture. The newer, very low-dose estrogen oral contraceptives, which tend to suppress menstruation, may also be associated with bone loss and fracture. Men treated with androgen deprivation therapy, such as prostate cancer treatment with Lupron, are also at risk of bone loss and fracture.

DIABETES MELLITUS

The incidence of diabetes continues to climb worldwide. Type I and Type II diabetes mellitus (DM) are associated with osteoporosis and fracture. The increased risk seems due to the direct effect of the metabolic syndrome associated with DM on the skeleton, the complications of DM, and an increased risk of falls. Patients with DM may have retinopathy, affecting vision and causing an increased risk of falls. Neuropathy may cause a person to be less active and to have an increased risk of falls. Data from the Iowa Women's Health Study suggested that women with Type 1 DM are 12 times more likely to sustain hip fractures than women without DM and that women with Type 2 DM have a 1.7-fold increased risk of sustaining hip fractures despite maintaining a normal bone mass.[34] A report on DM and the risk of hip fracture in the Singapore Chinese Health Study demonstrated that DM and duration of disease had a direct effect on hip-fracture risk.[35] The primary cause of loss of bone mass seems to be a low bone-formation rate and low bone turnover.[36] High glucose levels in vitro result in osteoblastic dysfunction. It is anticipated that children with Type 1 DM would never reach expected peak bone mass.

Also, DM is associated with increased adiposity in bone marrow. Increased bone marrow adiposity has been associated with osteoporosis in certain conditions, such as aging, immobility, and glucocorticoid use. It is better understood that adipogenesis and osteogenesis are interconnected.

Thiazolidinedione (TZD) use has increasingly been shown to be a cause of bone loss and increased fracture risk. This group of drugs is commonly used to treat osteoporosis. A recent study demonstrated a 39% higher incidence of fractures in men and women exposed to a TZD compared with controls.[37,38]

CUSHING SYNDROME

Cushing syndrome involves endogenous production of cortisol by adrenal hyperplasia or by an adrenal adenoma or malignancy. One of the myriad associated clinical features is increased bone resorption, osteoporosis, and increased risk of fracture. In patients suspected of having Cushing syndrome, 24-hour urine cortisol level is checked. If elevated, the adrenal glands are imaged. Traditionally, large, functioning adenomas are removed, thus treating the underlying condition. More recent studies have focused on subclinical Cushing syndrome (SCS) due to adrenal incidentaloma (the autonomous hypersecretion of a small amount of cortisol, which is not enough to cause clinically-evident disease). Traditionally, these patients are followed on a regular basis, but low-grade chronic cortisol secretion could have negative health effects, especially on the skeleton. One randomized, prospective study evaluating patients with SCS compared observation to laparoscopic removal of adenomas. Patients who underwent surgery had improved control of hypertension, hyperlipidemia, obesity, and DM, but there were no changes in bone parameters in patients with osteoporosis.[39] A retrospective study looking at a similar group of patients had similar findings.[40]

Patients with Cushing syndrome should have a baseline bone-density test and should be treated for osteoporosis or osteopenia with an appropriate antiresorptive or anabolic agent as clinically indicated. A recent study evaluated whether patients with SCS would benefit from antiresorptive therapy.[41] Patients with SCS due to an adrenal incidentaloma and osteoporosis/osteopenia were randomized to receive clodronate or placebo for 12 months. Patients who received clodronate had increased lumbar BMD values, preserved bone mass in the femoral neck, decreased bone-turnover markers, stabilized vertebral fracture index, and decreased subjective back pain compared with controls. The control group had a slight loss in BMD, and bone-turnover markers did not change significantly. Taken together, patients with SCS should have a bone-health evaluation, and treatment with an antiresorptive or anabolic agent should be considered strongly.

HYPERPROLACTINEMIA

Elevated prolactin levels are associated with bone loss and osteoporotic fractures.[42] In has been demonstrated that treatment of hyperprolactinemia with bromocriptine restores normal values of bone-formation and bone-resorption markers.[43] Many medical conditions and medications can cause hyperprolactinemia (**Box 1**). Much data suggest that many antipsychotics, such as risperidone, haloperidol, and chlorpromazine, are associated with lower bone density in treated patients.[44] Screening patients at risk of hyperprolactinemia seems reasonable to help maximize bone health.

CKD MINERAL BONE DISORDER

CKD mineral bone disorder (MBD) has been designed to replace the term renal osteo-dystrophy (ROD) as knowledge about bone disease in patients with CKD has emerged, and it is now known that there are many facets to bone disease in these patients. ROD refers to skeletal pathology and CKD-MBD refers to the entire spectrum of mineral metabolism, cardiovascular, and skeletal complications of CKD.[45] The earliest histologic abnormalities of bone in CKD-MBD are seen after a fairly mild reduction in the glomerular filtration rate (creatinine clearance between 40 and 70 mL/min). Often, PTH and fibroblast growth factor 23 (FGF-23) levels may be elevated before changes in serum phosphorus, calcitriol, or calcium levels are seen.[46] In CKD, if hyperparathyroidism is prevented or treated, a low-turnover osteodystrophy, the adynamic bone disorder, is seen. By the time the creatinine clearance is less than 15 mL/min, skeletal pathology is found in nearly all patients.[47] Decreased osteoblastic function and bone formation rates is seen in CKD. Abnormalities in vitamin D, calcium, and phosphate levels stimulate PTH, causing a state of high bone-turnover and result-ing ultimately in osteitis fibrosis.

There are many causes of secondary hyperparathyroidism in CKD. Hyperphospha-temia is a result of there being fewer nephrons available for filtration of phosphorus. Consequently, there is an elevation of PTH and FGF-23, resulting in increased phos-phate excretion by remaining nephrons and an attempt at maintaining a normal

---

Box 1
Common causes of hyperprolactinemia

Physiologic secretion

Pituitary tumors

Pituitary granulomatous process

Acromegaly

Chronic renal disease

Hypothyroidism

Cirrhosis

Seizures

Drug-induced secretion

    Dopamine receptor blockers

    Dopamine synthesis inhibitors

    Catecholamine depletors

    Opiates

    H_2 receptor antagonists

    Imipramines

    Serotonin-reuptake inhibitors

    Calcium channel blockers

    Estrogens/antiandrogens

phosphorus level. A direct effect of phosphorus on the parathyroid glands contributes to parathyroid gland hyperplasia. Hyperphosphatemia is also a signaling mechanism for heterotopic mineralization of the vasculature in CKD.

Because of progressive loss of nephrons, there is less calcitriol (1, 25 vitamin D) production by the proximal tubular 25-hydroxy cholecalciferol 1α-hydroxylase.[48] Also, the increased phosphate load leads to calcitriol deficiency, resulting in decreased intestinal calcium absorption and hypocalcemia. In advanced kidney disease, low calcitriol levels lead to tissue VDRs, especially on the parathyroid glands,[49] resulting in the synthesis of PTH.

In CKD, hypocalcemia develops because of decreased calcium absorption, resulting in hyperparathyroidism. Expression of the calcium receptor has been shown to be decreased by calcitriol deficiency and stimulated by calcitriol administration. The decreased number of calcium-sensing receptors may explain the relative insensitivity of parathyroid gland to calcium in patients undergoing dialysis.

In summary, hyperphosphatemia, calcitriol deficiency, and hypocalcemia all contribute to secondary hyperparathyroidism in CKD. The parathyroid glands develop nodular hyperplasia. Chronically elevated PTH levels are associated with active bone resorption and a high bone-turnover state.

ROD has several distinct features. Sustained excess of PTH results in a high bone-turnover state. There is an abundance of osteoclasts, osteoblasts, and osteocytes. Collagen is laid down in a disorganized fashion resulting in woven bone. There is fibrosis in the peritrabecular and bone marrow space, increased osteoid volume, and possibly, low bone-turnover state that is marked by low rates of bone resorption and formation. There is a low mineralization rate. Bone is primarily lamellar. There can also be a mixed picture with defective mineralization caused by excess aluminum.

In ROD, there is usually a net loss of cortical and cancellous bone. Clinically, this commonly results in osteopenia and osteoporosis. The prevalence of osteoporosis in patients with CKD exceeds the prevalence in the general population.[50,51] Osteoporosis may be observed in CKD before dialysis is required for end-stage renal disease.[52] A recent report describes hypoparathyroidism and hypoalbuminemia as risk factors of hip fractures in hemodialysis patients.[53] Rapid rates of bone resorption result in hypercalcemia and hyperphosphatemia, which are associated with heterotopic mineralization, especially in the vasculature. In secondary hyperparathyroidism, bone formation can exceed bone resorption. This can result is osteosclerosis; unfortunately, the bone is often of poor quality, being primarily woven bone.

Defective mineralization can be seen when excess amounts of aluminum, iron, and lanthanum are administered. These substances accumulate on the mineralization front. Lanthanum is used as a phosphate binder. Less aluminum is used in the dialysate than in the past, which has reduced the incidence of aluminum toxicity. It is becoming clearer that bisphosphonate administration to patients with CKD may cause accumulation in bone for prolonged periods of time, also affecting mineralization.

Clinical Manifestations of CKD

Patients with ROD are at risk of vascular calcification; calcification can occur in the neointimal and arterial medial parts of the vessel wall, which can cause an increase in systolic blood pressure, widening of pulse pressure, and increase in pulse pressure velocity. These findings can result in left ventricular dysfunction, diastolic dysfunction, and coronary ischemia, which is most common in patients with advanced kidney disease. Preceding signs include hypocalcemia, hyperphosphatemia, and hyperparathyroidism. Physicians are much better at monitoring for and treating these complications than in the past.

Heterotopic calcification can occur in many areas. In the eye, it can cause band keratopathy in the sclera or "red-eye syndrome" in the conjunctiva. An abnormal calcium phosphate product contributes to soft tissue calcification. Calcific masses may be quite large, and if they are periarticular, joint function can be compromised. Calcification in the lung can cause restrictive lung disease. Calcification in the heart can cause arrhythmia or myocardial dysfunction. Calciphylaxis is characterized by calcification of the tunica media of the peripheral arteries. This induces painful, violaceous skin lesions that become necrotic and is often associated with death.

Patients with CKD often complain of vague bone pain, which may be diffuse or localized in the lower extremities and can be aggravated by weight-bearing and incapacitating. Involved bones can be tender. Joint pain can be acute and severe. In patients with pain, careful consideration should be given to fractures, given the poor bone quality and frequency of osteoporosis in this population. Patients with a low bone-turnover state and aluminum-related bone disease tend to have the most severe bone pain. Thoracic kyphosis can be seen with associated vertebral fractures.

Diagnosis

Because of the heterogeneity of ROD, the gold standard for identification of bone disease is bone biopsy. The Kidney Disease: Improving Global Outcomes recommendations suggest that ROD be characterized for rates of bone turnover, bone mass, and mineralization. PTH levels have been correlated with bone turnover in biopsy studies to estimate remodeling. It has been shown that all patients with serum PTH levels of 100 pg/mL or less have a low bone turnover.[54] Values of serum PTH greater than 500 pg/mL are 100% and 95% specific for high-dose turnover in patients maintained on hemodialysis and peritoneal dialysis, respectively.[54] For patients with serum PTH levels between 65 and 500 pg/mL, bone turnover is difficult to predict. There are certain risk factors that suggest a low bone-turnover state, such as diabetes, prior parathyroidectomy, aggressive vitamin D therapy, high calcium content in the dialysate, high doses of calcium-based phosphate binders, and peritoneal dialysis.

DEXA tends not to be very reliable in CKD because of sclerosis and poor bone quality. There can also be inaccuracy because of heterotopic ossification, which can falsely elevate the DEXA reading, especially of the lumbar spine. A recent report describes the insufficiencies of DEXA in hemodialysis patients and the need to include the appendicular skeleton in the analysis.[55] Studies on the use of quantitative computed tomography, micro-magnetic resonance imaging (MRI), and peripheral ultrasonography may prove useful in assessing bone density and strength in this population.

Prevention and Treatment

It is recommended that treatment of CKD-MBD begin when the creatinine clearance less than 60 mL/min per 1.73 m^2. This is when hyperphosphatemia and calcitriol deficiency begin. Patients are instructed on a protein-restricted diet, because protein-rich foods contain a considerable amount of phosphorus. Dialysis does remove phosphorus, but not as much as is ingested. Consequently, phosphate binders are prescribed. Common phosphate binders include calcium acetate, sevelamer, calcium carbonate, and lanthanum carbonate. Calcium citrate should be avoided, because it promotes intestinal aluminum absorption. Calcium-containing phosphate binders may cause hypercalcemia; they may suppress bone formation and promote vascular calcification. Sevelamer seems to cause less vascular calcification than calcium-containing phosphorus binders, but is more expensive. Long-term data on lanthanum is limited. Hypocalcemia can usually be corrected with control of serum phosphorus level and vitamin D therapy.

Vitamin D deficiency is common in CKD. Replacement of calcitriol with vitamin D analogs should be started in patients with CKD and is necessary in all dialysis patients. Vitamin D therapy helps control hyperparathyroidism. Oral calcitriol in doses of 0.25 to 0.5 µg/d can be used in patients with CKD not yet requiring dialysis. Hypercalcemia may enforce the adjustment of dietary and supplemental calcium. Intravenous vitamin analogs are also available and have largely replaced oral calcitriol in patients on dialysis.

Calcimimetics are agents that modulate the calcium-sensing receptor. This class of therapeutics can suppress PTH and lower serum calcium (Ca). Cinacalcet may increase the number of patients achieving a satisfactory Ca $\times$ PO$_4$ product, but it is not yet clear whether this has long-term benefits.[56] For patients with elevated PTH levels despite the aforementioned measures, parathyroidectomy remains an option, as it does for patients with persistent bone pain, pruritus, or extensive soft tissue calcification.

Treatment options for osteoporosis in late-stage CKD are otherwise quite limited. Bisphosphonates are generally not recommended for patients with CKD, because of the potential to contribute to an adynamic bone state and bone that is more fragile. A recent study looking at histology in patients with CKD who had received bisphosphonates demonstrated decreased cancellous bone mass, decreased osteoid surface, decreased osteoid thickness, and low or low-normal osteoclastic/osteoblastic interface; these findings were suggestive of an adynamic bone state and the investigators concluded that the use of bisphosphonates should not be recommended in CKD. For patients with early CKD, antiresorptive and anabolic agents remain an option. PTH is not an option in patients with late-stage CKD and hyperparathyroidism.

Glucocorticoid-Induced Osteoporosis

Glucocorticoid-induced osteoporosis (GIO) is the second-most common cause of osteoporosis and the most common cause of drug-induced osteoporosis.[57,58] Many patients receive glucocorticoids for many reasons and unfortunately, many health care providers are not diligent in screening and treating patients on glucocorticoids for bone health. It is best to know the BMD of a patient before initiating glucocorticoids. Unfortunately, this is not always possible. Health care providers should attempt to define the risk factors of osteoporosis before initiating glucocorticoid therapy. The most bone loss is seen within the first 3 months of glucocorticoid therapy. Bone loss is actually biphasic, with a reduction in BMD of 6% to 12% within the first year and a slower annual loss thereafter.[59] It is clear that BMD is not a surrogate for fracture. For the same BMD, a patient on glucocorticoids is more prone to fractures than one not on glucocorticoids. GIO affects both cortical and cancellous bone, but there is a greater risk of fracture of cancellous (trabecular) bone. The higher the dose of glucocorticoid, the greater the risk of fracture.

Pathophysiology

Histomorphometric studies of patients on glucocorticoids have shown reduced numbers of osteoblasts on cancellous bone.[57] Glucocorticoids suppress formation of osteoblasts resulting in a decreased bone formation rate. Osteoclast numbers in patients receiving chronic glucocorticoids are within the normal range or slightly increased. Studies show that glucocorticoids result in the rapid loss of BMD caused by an imbalance in osteoblast and osteoclast numbers. Glucocorticoids reduce the number of osteoblast and osteoclast precursors but also increase the lifespan of osteoclasts.[60] Bisphosphonates are unable to prevent this process, which may explain why they are not as effective in GIO compared with postmenopausal osteoporosis or male osteoporosis.[61] At one point, it was thought that a significant cause of GIO was a hypogonadal state because of decreased production of sex steroids; studies have proven that this is not a significant cause of GIO. There was also a sense that GIO was caused from hyperparathyroidism, which has also been disproven. Glucocorticoids, early in their use, downregulate OPG production while the production of RANKL is increased,[62,63] This may help to explain why there is a rapid onset of loss of bone when glucocorticoid therapy is initiated.

Treatment

It is critical that anyone prescribing glucocorticoids consider the bone health of the patient. Risk factors of fracture should be assessed. The WHO has defined the Fracture Risk Assessment Tool (FRAX; http://www.sheffield.ac.uk/FRAX/), which helps define the risk of fracture in a given patient over the next 10 years. The FRAX analysis does ask if the patient is on glucocorticoids. The bone density result is also necessary to complete the FRAX analysis. This should be updated, if not completed, in the last 1 to 2 years. The FRAX analysis recommends treatment if the overall risk of fracture over the next 10 years is 20% or greater and of hip fracture, 3% or greater. Alternatively, health care practitioners may opt to treat all patients with osteoporosis on glucocorticoids and a significant number with osteopenia depending on other risk factors. A general rule is to treat all patients who are to be on glucocorticoids for 3 months or more or those who are to be on frequent courses of glucocorticoids. Low-dose thiazide diuretics can help reduce the hypercalciuria seen in patients on glucocorticoids.

All patients should be prescribed calcium and vitamin D to correct vitamin D deficiency and secondary hyperparathyroidism. A weight-bearing exercise regimen is particularly important, because this benefits bone health and helps combat muscle atrophy seen with glucocorticoid use. Clinicians should always try to prescribe the lowest dose possible for the shortest duration possible to control the inflammatory process. Bisphosphonates have been shown to reduce the risk of fractures in patients on glucocorticoids; in select patients on glucocorticoids, the use of a bisphosphonate is a reasonable option.[64] Care should be taken to avoid oversuppression in patients on lower dose glucocorticoids for a prolonged time, because these patients may be at greater risk of osteonecrosis of the jaw. Bone markers of resorption, such as the urine N-telopeptide (NTX) or serum C-telopeptide (CTX), may prove useful in deciding on duration of bisphosphonate use in patients on bisphosphonates and glucocorticoids.

PTH has been shown to be superior to bisphosphonates in preventing GIO. Glucocorticoids are known to reduce osteoblastic function. PTH is an anabolic agent and promotes osteoblastic function. Women with various rheumatologic conditions being treated with hormone replacement therapy were randomized to receive teriparatide and hormone therapy or teriparatide alone.[39] Patients on teriparatide had a 12% increase in sine BMD by DEXA and a smaller increase in femoral neck BMD. In an 18-month trial of teriparatide versus alendronate for GIO, patients treated with teriparatide had an increase of 7.2% at the spine and 3.8% in the total hip compared with 3.4% and 2.4%, respectively, seen in the alendronate-treated patients.[65] There were also fewer vertebral fractures seen in the teriparatide-treated group.

GLUCOCORTICOID-INDUCED OSTEONECROSIS

This tends to be an unpredictable and devastating consequence of glucocorticoid use. Patients experience often acute pain in a joint. MRI initially reveals bone marrow edema, most commonly in the femoral neck. The involved area of bone can go on to collapse, and the patient may require a total joint replacement. Almost any joint can be involved, but large joints are most commonly affected. It has long been thought that this process was the result of fat emboli, microvascular tamponade of blood vessels of involved bone by fat or fluid retention, and nonhealing stress fractures. More recent data suggest that this process is the result of osteocyte apoptosis.[60,66]

SUMMARY

As the population ages, the amount of metabolic bone disease and number of fractures will increase. It is imperative that health care providers screen and treat patients at risk of metabolic bone disease. There is much research ongoing in this field and the number of treatment options will greatly expand. Focusing on ways to maximize the development of the fetal skeleton to improve peak bone mass, such as improving maternal vitamin D levels during pregnancy, may best address the treatment of osteoporosis and osteomalacia for the entire population.

REFERENCES

1. Zaidi M, Davies TF, Zallone A, et al. Thyroid-stimulating hormone, thyroid hormones, and bone loss. Curr Osteoporos Rep 2009;7(2):47–52.
2. Baqi L, Payer J, Killinger Z, et al. Thyrotropin versus thyroid hormone in regulating bone density and turnover in premenopausal women. Endocr Regul 2010;44(2): 57–63.
3. Abe E, Sun L, Mechanick J, et al. Bone loss in thyroid disease: role of low TSH and high thyroid hormone. Ann N Y Acad Sci 2007;1116:383–91.
4. Faber J, Perrild H, Johansen JS. Bone Gla protein and sex hormone-binding globulin in nontoxic goiter: parameters for metabolic status at the tissue level. J Clin Endocrinol Metab 1990;70(1):49–55.
5. Schneider DL, Barrett-Connor EL, Morton DJ. Thyroid hormone use and bone mineral density in elderly men. Arch Intern Med 1995;155(18):2005–7.
6. Rosen HN, Moses AC, Gundberg C, et al. Therapy with parenteral pamidronate prevents thyroid hormone-induced bone turnover in humans. J Clin Endocrinol Metab 1993;77(3):664–9.
7. Bilezikian JP, Silverberg SJ. Clinical practice. asymptomatic primary hyperparathyroidism. N Engl J Med 2004;350(17):1746–51.
8. Silverberg SJ, Shane E, Jacobs TP, et al. A 10-year prospective study of primary hyperparathyroidism with or without parathyroid surgery. N Engl J Med 1999; 341(17):1249–55.
9. Binkley N, Ramamurthy R, Krueger D. Low vitamin D status: definition, prevalence, consequences, and correction. Endocrinol Metab Clin North Am 2010; 39(2):287–301, table of contents.
10. Khan A, Grey A, Shoback D. Medical management of asymptomatic primary hyperparathyroidism: proceedings of the third international workshop. J Clin Endocrinol Metab 2009;94(2):373–81.
11. Mosekilde L. Primary hyperparathyroidism and the skeleton. Clin Endocrinol (Oxf) 2008;69(1):1–19.
12. Unverdi S, Ozturk MA, Inal S, et al. Idiopathic hypoparathyroidism mimicking diffuse idiopathic skeletal hyperostosis. J Clin Rheumatol 2009;15(7):361–2.
13. Rubin MR, Bilezikian JP. Hypoparathyroidism: clinical features, skeletal microstructure and parathyroid hormone replacement. Arq Bras Endocrinol Metabol 2010;54(2):220–6.

14. Rubin MR, Sliney J Jr, McMahon DJ, et al. Therapy of hypoparathyroidism with intact parathyroid hormone. Osteoporos Int 2010;21(11):1927–34.

15. Lips P. Relative value of 25(OH)D and 1,25(OH)2D measurements. J Bone Miner Res 2007;22(11):1668–71.

16. Bischoff-Ferrari HA, Willett WC, Wong JB, et al. Fracture prevention with vitamin D supplementation: a meta-analysis of randomized controlled trials. JAMA 2005; 293(18):2257–64.

17. Boonen S, Lips P, Bouillon R, et al. Need for additional calcium to reduce the risk of hip fracture with vitamin d supplementation: evidence from a comparative metaanalysis of randomized controlled trials. J Clin Endocrinol Metab 2007; 92(4):1415–23.

18. Carpenter TO, DeLucia MC, Zhang JH, et al. A randomized controlled study of effects of dietary magnesium oxide supplementation on bone mineral content in healthy girls. J Clin Endocrinol Metab 2006;91(12):4866–72.

19. Christakos S, Dhawan P, Peng X, et al. New insights into the function and regulation of vitamin D target proteins. J Steroid Biochem Mol Biol 2007;103(3–5): 405–10.

20. Goltzman D. Use of genetically modified mice to examine the skeletal anabolic activity of vitamin D. J Steroid Biochem Mol Biol 2007;103(3–5):587–91.

21. Lips P. Which circulating level of 25-hydroxyvitamin D is appropriate? J Steroid Biochem Mol Biol 2004;89–90(1–5):611–4.

22. Whyte MP. Atypical femoral fractures, bisphosphonates, and adult hypophosphatasia. J Bone Miner Res 2009;24(6):1132–4.

23. Prie D, Huart V, Bakouh N, et al. Nephrolithiasis and osteoporosis associated with hypophosphatemia caused by mutations in the type 2a sodium-phosphate cotransporter. N Engl J Med 2002;347(13):983–91.

24. Rude RK, Gruber HE, Norton HJ, et al. Bone loss induced by dietary magnesium reduction to 10% of the nutrient requirement in rats is associated with increased release of substance P and tumor necrosis factor-alpha. J Nutr 2004;134(1): 79–85.

25. Khosla S, Riggs BL. Pathophysiology of age-related bone loss and osteoporosis. Endocrinol Metab Clin North Am 2005;34(4):1015–30, xi.

26. Hughes DE, Dai A, Tiffee JC, et al. Estrogen promotes apoptosis of murine osteoclasts mediated by TGF-beta. Nat Med 1996;2(10):1132–6.

27. Manolagas SC. Birth and death of bone cells: Basic regulatory mechanisms and implications for the pathogenesis and treatment of osteoporosis. Endocr Rev 2000;21(2):115–37.

28. Chow J, Tobias JH, Colston KW, et al. Estrogen maintains trabecular bone volume in rats not only by suppression of bone resorption but also by stimulation of bone formation. J Clin Invest 1992;89(1):74–8.

29. Qu Q, Perala-Heape M, Kapanen A, et al. Estrogen enhances differentiation of osteoblasts in mouse bone marrow culture. Bone 1998;22(3):201–9.

30. Khastgir G, Studd J, Holland N, et al. Anabolic effect of estrogen replacement on bone in postmenopausal women with osteoporosis: histomorphometric evidence in a longitudinal study. J Clin Endocrinol Metab 2001;86(1):289–95.

31. Hofbauer LC, Khosla S, Dunstan CR, et al. Estrogen stimulates gene expression and protein production of osteoprotegerin in human osteoblastic cells. Endocrinology 1999;140(9):4367–70.

32. Slemenda CW, Longcope C, Zhou L, et al. Sex steroids and bone mass in older men. positive associations with serum estrogens and negative associations with androgens. J Clin Invest 1997;100(7):1755–9.

33. Khosla S, Melton LJ 3rd, Atkinson EJ, et al. Relationship of serum sex steroid levels to longitudinal changes in bone density in young versus elderly men. J Clin Endocrinol Metab 2001;86(8):3555–61.

34. Nicodemus KK, Folsom AR, Anderson KE. Menstrual history and risk of hip fractures in postmenopausal women. the iowa women's health study. Am J Epidemiol 2001;153(3):251–5.

35. Koh WP, Wang R, Ang LW, et al. Diabetes and risk of hip fracture in the Singapore Chinese Health Study. Diabetes Care 2010;33(8):1766–70.

36. Bouillon R, Bex M, Van Herck E, et al. Influence of age, sex, and insulin on osteoblast function: osteoblast dysfunction in diabetes mellitus. J Clin Endocrinol Metab 1995;80(4):1194–202.

37. Aubert RE, Herrera V, Chen W, et al. Rosiglitazone and pioglitazone increase fracture risk in women and men with type 2 diabetes. Diabetes Obes Metab 2010; 12(8):716–21.

38. Vestergaard P. Bone metabolism in type 2 diabetes and role of thiazolidinediones. Curr Opin Endocrinol Diabetes Obes 2009;16(2):125–31.

39. Toniato A, Merante-Boschin I, Opocher G, et al. Surgical versus conservative management for subclinical Cushing syndrome in adrenal incidentalomas: a prospective randomized study. Ann Surg 2009;249(3):388–91.

40. Guerrieri M, Campagnacci R, Patrizi A, et al. Primary adrenal hypercortisolism: minimally invasive surgical treatment or medical therapy? A retrospective study with long-term follow-up evaluation. Surg Endosc 2010;24(10):2542–6.

41. Tauchmanova L, Guerra E, Pivonello R, et al. Weekly clodronate treatment prevents bone loss and vertebral fractures in women with subclinical Cushing's syndrome. J Endocrinol Invest 2009;32(5):390–4.

42. Naliato EC, Farias ML, Braucks GR, et al. Prevalence of osteopenia in men with prolactinoma. J Endocrinol Invest 2005;28(1):12–7.

43. Shaarawy M, El-Dawakhly AS, Mosaad M, et al. Biomarkers of bone turnover and bone mineral density in hyperprolactinemic amenorrheic women. Clin Chem Lab Med 1999;37(4):433–8.

44. Renn JH, Yang NP, Chou P. Effects of plasma magnesium and prolactin on quantitative ultrasound measurements of heel bone among schizophrenic patients. BMC Musculoskelet Disord 2010;11:35.

45. Moe S, Drueke T, Cunningham J, et al. Kidney Disease: Improving Global Outcomes (KDIGO). Definition, evaluation, and classification of renal osteodystrophy: a position statement from kidney disease: Improving global outcomes (KDIGO). Kidney Int 2006;69(11):1945–53.

46. Malluche HH, Ritz E, Lange HP, et al. Bone histology in incipient and advanced renal failure. Kidney Int 1976;9(4):355–62.

47. Malluche H, Faugere MC. Renal bone disease 1990: an unmet challenge for the nephrologist. Kidney Int 1990;38(2):193–211.

48. Goodman WG, Quarles LD. Development and progression of secondary hyperparathyroidism in chronic kidney disease: lessons from molecular genetics. Kidney Int 2008;74(3):276–88.

49. Naveh-Many T, Marx R, Keshet E, et al. Regulation of 1,25-dihydroxyvitamin D3 receptor gene expression by 1,25-dihydroxyvitamin D3 in the parathyroid in vivo. J Clin Invest 1990;86(6):1968–75.

50. Alem AM, Sherrard DJ, Gillen DL, et al. Increased risk of hip fracture among patients with end-stage renal disease. Kidney Int 2000;58(1):396–9.

51. Cunningham J, Sprague SM, Cannata-Andia J, et al. Osteoporosis work group. Osteoporosis in chronic kidney disease. Am J Kidney Dis 2004;43(3):566–71.

52. Rix M, Andreassen H, Eskildsen P, et al. Bone mineral density and biochemical markers of bone turnover in patients with predialysis chronic renal failure. Kidney Int 1999;56(3):1084–93.

53. Al Helal B, Su WS, Churchill DN, et al. Relative hypoparathyroidism and hypoalbuminemia are associated with hip fracture in hemodialysis patients. Clin Nephrol 2010;73(2):88–93.

54. Levey AS, Coresh J, Balk E, et al, National Kidney Foundation. National kidney foundation practice guidelines for chronic kidney disease: evaluation, classification, and stratification. Ann Intern Med 2003;139(2):137–47.

55. Orlic L, Crncevic Z, Pavlovic D, et al. Bone mineral densitometry in patients on hemodialysis: difference between genders and what to measure. Ren Fail 2010;32(3):300–8.

56. Block GA, Martin KJ, de Francisco AL, et al. Cinacalcet for secondary hyperparathyroidism in patients receiving hemodialysis. N Engl J Med 2004;350(15): 1516–25.

57. Weinstein RS. Glucocorticoid-induced osteoporosis. Rev Endocr Metab Disord 2001;2(1):65–73.

58. Canalis E, Mazziotti G, Giustina A, et al. Glucocorticoid-induced osteoporosis: pathophysiology and therapy. Osteoporos Int 2007;18(10):1319–28.

59. LoCascio V, Bonucci E, Imbimbo B, et al. Bone loss in response to long-term glucocorticoid therapy. Bone Miner 1990;8(1):39–51.

60. Weinstein RS, Nicholas RW, Manolagas SC. Apoptosis of osteocytes in glucocorticoid-induced osteonecrosis of the hip. J Clin Endocrinol Metab 2000;85(8): 2907–12.

61. Curtis JR, Westfall AO, Allison JJ, et al. Longitudinal patterns in the prevention of osteoporosis in glucocorticoid-treated patients. Arthritis Rheum 2005;52(8): 2485–94.

62. Hofbauer LC, Gori F, Riggs BL, et al. Stimulation of osteoprotegerin ligand and inhibition of osteoprotegerin production by glucocorticoids in human osteoblastic lineage cells: potential paracrine mechanisms of glucocorticoid-induced osteoporosis. Endocrinology 1999;140(10):4382–9.

63. Vidal NO, Brandstrom H, Jonsson KB, et al. Osteoprotegerin mRNA is expressed in primary human osteoblast-like cells: down-regulation by glucocorticoids. J Endocrinol 1998;159(1):191–5.

64. Adachi JD, Saag KG, Delmas PD, et al. Two-year effects of alendronate on bone mineral density and vertebral fracture in patients receiving glucocorticoids: a randomized, double-blind, placebo-controlled extension trial. Arthritis Rheum 2001;44(1):202–11.

65. Dempster DW. Bone histomorphometry in glucocorticoid-induced osteoporosis. J Bone Miner Res 1989;4(2):137–41.

66. Calder JD, Buttery L, Revell PA, et al. Apoptosis–a significant cause of bone cell death in osteonecrosis of the femoral head. J Bone Joint Surg Br 2004;86(8): 1209–13.

Rheumatic Manifestations of Diabetes Mellitus

Dorota Lebiedz-Odrobina, MD, Jonathan Kay, MD*

KEYWORDS

• Rheumatic manifestations • Diabetes mellitus
• Advanced glycation end products • Joint • Muscle
• Hand • Shoulder

Diabetes mellitus (DM) is a widespread chronic disease, the complications of which affect several different organ systems. According to the National Health and Nutrition Examination Survey (NHANES), the crude prevalence of DM was 9.3% during the period between 1999 and 2002, affecting 19.3 million individuals in the United States. The prevalence of diabetes increases with age, reaching 21.6% among individuals 65 years and older.[1] Type 1 DM results from an absolute deficiency of insulin due to auto-immune destruction of insulin-producing beta cells within the pancreas. Type 2 DM, which affects up to 95% of diabetics, is caused by resistance to insulin resulting in a relative deficiency of that hormone.[2]

Insulin resistance is a feature common to type 2 DM and the metabolic syndrome. To be diagnosed with the metabolic syndrome, a patient must have at least 3 of the following clinical features: hyperglycemia or receiving treatment for DM, hypercholes-terolemia, hypertriglyceridemia, abdominal obesity, and hypertension.[3] It remains unresolved as to whether the metabolic syndrome is simply a constellation of risk factors that predispose to developing type 2 DM and coronary artery disease or if it represents the clinical manifestations of a specific underlying pathophysiologic mechanism, such as insulin resistance.[4]

In contrast to the extensively studied microvascular and macrovascular complications, characterization of the musculoskeletal complications of DM is derived predominantly from observational studies. Several authors have attempted to classify the rheumatic manifestations of DM.[5–7] However, pathogenetic mechanisms for many of these conditions have not yet been elucidated; their association with DM is based largely on epidemiologic data.[5]

Rheumatology Division, Department of Medicine, University of Massachusetts School of Medicine, 55 Lake Avenue North, Worcester, MA 01655, USA
* Corresponding author. Rheumatology Center, UMass Memorial Medical Center, Memorial Campus, 119 Belmont Street, Worcester, MA 01605.
E-mail address: jonathan.kay@umassmemorial.org

Rheum Dis Clin N Am 36 (2010) 681–699
doi:10.1016/j.rdc.2010.09.008
0889-857X/10/$ – see front matter © 2010 Elsevier Inc. All rights reserved.

Although only diabetic muscle infarction (DMI) has been reported to occur exclusively among patients with DM, several other rheumatologic disorders have been observed more frequently among individuals with DM than in the general population. Limited joint mobility (LJM) and neuropathic osteoarthropathy have been reported in nondiabetic individuals, but each occurs predominantly among patients with DM. Musculoskeletal disorders of the upper extremity, such as shoulder adhesive capsulitis, Dupuytren's disease (DD) and stenosing flexor tenosynovitis, occur 2 to 4 times as often among diabetic patients than in the general population.[8,9]

Hyperuricemia and gout are associated with the metabolic syndrome, but a direct relationship between these conditions and type 2 DM has not yet been established. Associations between type 2 DM and other musculoskeletal conditions, such as pseudogout or diffuse idiopathic skeletal hyperostosis (DISH), have not been proven. In this article, the authors discuss those rheumatic disorders that have been associated with DM or the metabolic syndrome and potential pathophysiologic relationships that might link these conditions (**Box 1**).

UPPER EXTREMITY MANIFESTATIONS OF DM
Limited Joint Mobility (Diabetic Cheiroarthropathy)

Hand stiffness as a complication of DM was first described in 1957 by Lundbaek in 5 adults with insulin-dependent DM[10] and subsequently in 1974 by Rosenbloom in 3 adolescents with type 1 DM.[11] The term *cheiroarthropathy* (derived from the Greek word *cheiros*, meaning hand) also has been used to describe this condition; however, use of the term *arthropathy* is inaccurate, because the pathologic process involves periarticular structures, not the joint itself.

Rosenbloom and colleagues[11] described 3 adolescents with type 1 DM who had flexion contractures involving several fingers and thickened, tight, and waxy skin predominantly over the dorsal aspect of the metacarpophalangeal, proximal, and

---

Box 1
Rheumatic complications of DM

Conditions unique to DM

    Diabetic muscle infarction

Conditions occurring more frequently in DM

    Neuropathic arthropathy

    Limited joint mobility

    Stiff hand syndrome

    Dupuytren's disease

    Stenosing flexor tenosynovitis (trigger finger)

    Shoulder capsulitis

    Calcific shoulder periarthritis

    Carpal tunnel syndrome

Conditions sharing risk factors of DM and metabolic syndrome

    Diffuse idiopathic skeletal hyperostosis

    Gout

    Osteoarthritis

distal interphalangeal joints of their fingers. They also had limited range of motion of large joints, such as the wrists, elbows, knees, and ankles, and of the spine. Also, these patients had short stature, delayed sexual maturation, and retinopathy or nephropathy, the diabetic microvascular complications of DM. Typically, the skin changes of LJM begin around the metacarpophalangeal and proximal interphalangeal joints of the little finger and progress medially to involve other digits and distally to involve the distal interphalangeal joints. LJM usually is painless and only mildly disabling.[12,13]

The clinical presentation of stiff hands in the adult diabetic patients described by Lundbaek[10] differed from that in the adolescents described by Rosenbloom.[11] The adult diabetics experienced paresthesias in their hands, followed by incapacitating pain that was exacerbated by activity. These patients also had stiff, hardened skin on their fingers and on the palms of their hands. A characteristic feature among these adults was the presence of arterial calcifications on plain radiographs. Histologic examination of skin demonstrated a paucity of elastic fibers. Rosenbloom proposed that this clinical entity is distinct from that which he observed in adolescents, and he named it the *stiff hand syndrome*.[13]

The prevalence of LJM ranges between 30% and 58% among patients with type 1 DM and between 45% and 76% among those with type 2 DM, as compared with between only 4% and 20% among individuals without DM.[14–18] The thickened, tightened, and waxy quality of skin on the fingers, the dorsum of the hands, and the forearms has been observed without LJM being present in 34% of diabetic patients.[19]

LJM is diagnosed based on the presence of characteristic findings on physical examination. The inability to appose the palmar surfaces of the hands and fingers with the wrists dorsiflexed is called the *prayer sign*. An alternative method of testing for LJM, called the *table top sign*, is considered to have an abnormal result if the entire surface of the palm and fingers cannot make contact with a flat surface when patients lay their palms on a tabletop with the fingers spread apart. Limited mobility should be confirmed by demonstrating loss of passive extension of the proximal interphalangeal and metacarpophalangeal joints (<180° and 60°, respectively). Rosenbloom and colleagues[15] proposed a classification system to stage this condition based on the type and number of joints involved (**Table 1**).

Several cross-sectional studies have correlated the presence of LJM with age and duration of DM.[14,20,21] Patients with type 1 DM and LJM were observed to have a higher incidence of retinopathy and nephropathy than those without LJM, even when adjusted for the confounding effect of duration of DM.[15,20,22] Type 2 diabetics with LJM also had a higher incidence of retinopathy and nephropathy and a greater

Table 1 Classification of LJM	
No limitation	Equivocal or unilateral findings
Mild limitation	Involvement of one or two interphalangeal joints, one large joint, or only the metacarpophalangeal joints bilaterally
Moderate limitation	Involvement of three or more interphalangeal joints or one finger joint and one large joint bilaterally
Severe limitation	Moderate limitation combined with cervical spine involvement or obvious hand deformity at rest

Data from Rosenbloom AL, Silverstein JH, Lezotte DC, et al. Limited joint mobility in childhood diabetes mellitus indicates increased risk for microvascular disease. N Engl J Med 1981;305(4):191–4.

requirement for insulin therapy, but no difference in hemoglobin A_{1c} (HbA_{1c}) levels, compared with those without LJM.[16] However, subsequent prospective studies failed to identify LJM as a predictor of the development of diabetic microvascular complications or the presence of microvascular complications as a predictor of developing cheiroarthropathy.[18,23,24] In contrast, the risk of developing macrovascular complications was increased among patients with type 2 DM and LJM, with 3- and 4-fold increased relative risks of developing coronary artery disease and cerebrovascular disease, respectively, even after controlling for age, duration of DM, and glycemic control.[25]

Inadequate glycemic control influences the progression of LJM among patients with type 1 DM.[26,27] Higher levels of HbA_{1c} were observed among patients with type 2 DM and LJM or shoulder adhesive capsulitis, suggesting that poor glycemic control might also contribute to developing these musculoskeletal conditions in type 2 DM.[28] However, other studies have failed to demonstrate an association between glycemic control and the presence of LJM.[16,18,23,29] The onset of hyperglycemia has been estimated to occur at least 4 to 7 years before type 2 DM is diagnosed; diabetic complications, such as retinopathy, already may be present when the clinical diagnosis is made.[30] Thus, longstanding hyperglycemia before the diagnosis of DM could also predispose to developing LJM. HbA_{1c} determinations from the period after initiation of glucose-lowering therapy might not reflect earlier prolonged hyperglycemia, especially among patients with type 2 DM, which could account for the apparent lack of correlation between laboratory measures of glycemic control and musculoskeletal manifestations of DM.

An observational study demonstrated a 4-fold decrease in the prevalence of LJM among children with type 1 DM, comparing the period between 1976 and 1978 with 1998.[31] Another study assessing the prevalence of LJM among adults with type 1 DM attending an endocrinology clinic in the United Kingdom also showed a statistically significant decrease in the prevalence of LJM from 43% during the period between 1981 and 1982 to 23% in 2002. The investigators hypothesized that implementation of an intensive glycemic control regimen accounted for the decreased prevalence of LJM. Although HbA_{1c} levels did not correlate with the presence of LJM, there was a trend toward a lower prevalence of LJM among patients with HbA_{1c} level less than 7%.[29]

Nonsteroidal anti-inflammatory drug and physical therapy remain the primary therapeutic modalities for patients with LJM. Increased range of motion and improved strength of finger flexion and extension has been reported in 3 diabetic patients with LJM who were treated with the hydantoin aldose reductase inhibitor, sorbinil[32]; however, clinical studies of sorbinil were stopped because of significant adverse effects, including adult respiratory distress syndrome, epidermic necrolysis, and Stevens-Johnson syndrome.[33]

Stenosing Flexor Tenosynovitis (Trigger Finger)

Stenosing flexor tenosynovitis typically presents with locking (or "triggering") of fingers in flexion, extension, or both, most commonly involving the thumb, middle, and ring fingers. In this condition, fibrosis and thickening of the tendon sheath, usually where it passes through a pulley or over a bony prominence, restricts movement of the flexor tendon within its tendon sheath. Tendon swelling distal to the site of constriction causes pain and difficulty flexing and extending the digit smoothly as the swollen segment of tendon passes through the narrowed space. Typically, this is followed by more severe symptoms of catching and, eventually, locking of involved fingers in flexion or extension.[34]

The prevalence of stenosing flexor tenosynovitis ranges between 5% and 36% among patients with type 1 and 2 DM, as compared with 2% in the general population.[9,35] The occurrence of trigger finger correlates significantly with duration of DM but not with glycemic control.[35] Compared with nondiabetics, patients with DM are more likely to have multiple fingers involved simultaneously by stenosing flexor tenosynovitis.[34,36]

Treatment of stenosing flexor tenosynovitis includes modification of activities to avoid triggering of digits, nonsteroidal anti-inflammatory drug therapy, splinting, corticosteroid injection into the tendon sheath, and surgical release.[37] Corticosteroid injection is less successful among patients with type 1 or 2 DM than with nondiabetics; systemic absorption of the depot corticosteroid occasionally can perturb glycemic control.[38,39] Patients with multiple digit involvement more often require surgical release to relieve symptoms.[40,41]

Dupuytren's Disease

DD is characterized by thickening of the palmar fascia, palmar or digital nodules, skin tethering, pretendinous bands, and flexion contractures of the fingers. Its presentation among patients with DM differs slightly from that in the general population. Among diabetics, DD most often involves the middle and ring fingers rather than the ring and little fingers, as in nondiabetics, and less often results in palmar contractures.[36,42]

DD is more prevalent among diabetics, affecting between 16% and 42%, than in the general population.[8,9,36,42] Among diabetics, DD occurs equally in both genders, whereas it occurs more often among men in the non-DM population.[13] However, among diabetics, severe DD and development of finger contractures is seen more often in men than women.[36,42] Because DD occurring in diabetic patients seldom requires surgical treatment, no significant association between DD and DM was identified in a large retrospective study of 2919 patients who had been referred for surgical treatment.[43]

Similar to LJM, the prevalence of DD among diabetics is higher with older age and longer duration of DM.[36,42] In cross-sectional studies, DD has been associated independently of age or duration of DM with the presence of retinopathy among patients with type 1 DM[20] and of severe retinopathy among patients with type 2 DM.[21] In a prospective study, the incidence of DD was higher among diabetic patients with hypertension and the microangiopathic complications of retinopathy, nephropathy, and neuropathy. However, when logistic regression analysis controlled for the confounding effects of age and duration of DM, the presence of DD no longer predicted the development of hypertension or of diabetic microangiopathic complications.[44]

Intralesional corticosteroid injections and surgery followed by hand therapy have been the standard treatments for DD. Recently, injecting the thickened palmar fascia with collagenase from *Clostridium histolyticum* has been developed as a nonsurgical approach to treating DD. In a prospective, randomized, placebo-controlled trial of 308 patients with DD, 6.5% of whom had DM, up to 3 collagenase injections significantly reduced fixed flexion contractures and significantly improved finger-joint range of motion; there were no recurrences of DD after up to 90 days of follow-up. Only 3 serious adverse events were reported in this study, including 2 tendon ruptures and 1 case of complex regional pain syndrome.[45] Although expensive, collagenase injection provides an alternative to surgical treatment of DD.

Adhesive Capsulitis of the Shoulder (Shoulder Periarthritis, Frozen Shoulder Syndrome)

Adhesive capsulitis usually presents as painful progressive restriction of range of shoulder motion, especially on abduction and external rotation. Its natural history can be divided into 3 phases: pain, stiffness, and recovery. The length of the recovery phase depends on the duration of the stiffness phase, with symptoms lasting for an average of 30 months.[46] The term *frozen shoulder* was first used to describe this condition in 1934 by Codman.[47] In 1945, Naviaser used the term *adhesive capsulitis* to describe the same entity.[48]

Adhesive capsulitis of the shoulder occurs more commonly among diabetics. The prevalence of shoulder periarthritis among diabetics ranges from 10% to 29% and is about 5-fold that in the general population.[14,23,49,50] In a cross-sectional study of 294 patients with type 1 DM and 134 patients with type 2 DM, the prevalence of shoulder adhesive capsulitis was 10% and 22%, respectively.[23] Shoulder adhesive capsulitis was more likely to develop in older individuals with either type of DM and in those with longer duration of disease among patients with type 1 DM. The apparent lack of association between shoulder adhesive capsulitis and disease duration in type 2 DM could be explained by the years of hyperglycemia that typically precede the diagnosis of type 2 DM. After controlling for the effects of age and disease duration, shoulder adhesive capsulitis is found to be associated with the presence of autonomic neuropathy among individuals with either type of DM and with myocardial infarction among those with type 1 DM. However, the presence of shoulder adhesive capsulitis did not correlate significantly with HbA_{1c} levels among patients with either type of DM.

An increased incidence of LJM among diabetic patients with shoulder adhesive capsulitis has been observed in some studies[23,50] but not confirmed in others.[14] Mean HbA_{1c} levels may be significantly higher among those diabetic patients with both shoulder and hand involvement than among those with no upper extremity problems,[51] which reflects the documented association between longstanding hyperglycemia and the development of LJM.

In idiopathic adhesive capsulitis, the joint capsule is thickened and adheres to the head of the humerus, thereby reducing the volume of the glenohumeral joint. Histologic and immunocytochemical examination of the joint capsule demonstrates proliferation of fibroblasts and transformation of some to myofibroblasts, which produce excess amounts of types I and III collagen, with subsequent contraction of the joint capsule that results in pain and stiffness. These findings are similar to DD of the hand.[52] In both conditions, expression of fibrogenic growth factors, matrix metalloproteinases (MMPs), and their inhibitors was increased, but expression of the proinflammatory cytokines interleukin (IL)-1β and tumor necrosis factor (TNF)-α and of TNF-β was lower in joint capsule tissue obtained from patients with adhesive capsulitis than in DD. This correlates with the histologic observation of relatively hypocellular, dense fibrous tissue with only a few mature fibroblasts, suggesting fibrosis rather than an active inflammatory process. In adhesive capsulitis, the lower expression of MMP-14, which plays a role in remodeling, could explain slow resolution of fibrosis.[53]

Analgesics, physical therapy, and intra-articular corticosteroid injections are first-line therapy during the initial painful phase of shoulder adhesive capsulitis. In a prospective study of a stretching-exercise program in 75 patients with idiopathic adhesive capsulitis including 8 with DM, 90% were satisfied with this treatment. However, the presence of DM was associated with an inferior outcome as evidenced by more pain, more restricted range of motion, and poorer function.[54] During the adhesive phase, physical therapy and operative treatments are typically used. Manipulation under anesthesia may be complicated by fracture, shoulder dislocation, tendon rupture, or neurologic injury. Arthroscopic capsular release has been an effective treatment modality for refractory shoulder adhesive capsulitis among diabetic patients.[55] In a study comparing arthroscopic capsular release in diabetic and nondiabetic patients, those with DM had poorer recovery of shoulder range-of-motion and function, but there was no significant difference in the duration of recovered range of motion or of complete pain relief.[56] Arthroscopic capsular release is preferred to open surgical release because of the reduced length of postoperative recovery.[57]

Pathogenesis of Limited Joint Mobility, Stenosing Flexor Tenosynovitis, Dupuytren's Disease, and Shoulder Adhesive Capsulitis

No single mechanism has been shown to account for the development of LJM and shoulder adhesive capsulitis, of stenosing flexor tenosynovitis, and of DD among patients with DM. However, the shared cause of these conditions seems to involve connective tissue deposition around joints, in tendon sheaths, and in the palmar fascia, respectively.[12] Although the pathogenesis of shoulder adhesive capsulitis in patients with DM has not been studied directly, its coexistence with LJM suggests a possible common mechanism. Histologic examination of skin from patients with LJM reveals thickening of the dermis and epidermis, accumulation of collagen and loss of skin appendages, increased nonenzymatic glycosylation, and cross-linkage of dermal collagen.[58] Accumulation of advanced glycation end products (AGEs) with cross-linking of collagen and other macromolecules has been proposed as a potential pathogenetic mechanism.[12]

AGEs are a heterogeneous group of compounds formed by a nonenzymatic reaction between the ketone group on reducing sugars and free amino groups on proteins, called the Maillard reaction. Initially, reversible Schiff bases and subsequently, more stable, covalently bound Amadori products (such as HbA_{1c}) are formed. These intermediate structures then undergo complex rearrangements to form the irreversibly cross-linked AGEs.[59] Lipids and nucleic acids exposed to reducing sugars also can form irreversible adducts with AGEs. Originally, all AGEs were believed to exhibit yellow-brown fluorescence and to cross-link macromolecules; however, several of the more recently identified AGEs, such as N-carboxymethyllysine and pyrraline, do not share these properties. Interaction of AGEs with the receptor for AGEs induces oxidative stress and inflammation and may promote thrombosis.[60]

The extent of AGE formation depends on the concentration of reducing sugars and the duration of time over which macromolecules are exposed to these sugars. Thus, long-lived macromolecules, such as extracellular matrix components in vascular endothelium, nerves, and connective tissue, are more likely to become modified with AGEs when exposed to high concentrations of glucose for prolonged periods of time. AGEs have been implicated in the development of both micro- and macrovascular complications of DM. The accumulation of AGEs in skin correlates with the presence of retinopathy, nephropathy, and LJM among patients with type 1 DM.[61] Because the Amadori product HbA_{1c} is an intermediate in the process of AGE formation, HbA_{1c} levels do not necessarily correlate with the extent of AGE modification of extracellular matrix macromolecules. Thus, despite the lack of correlation between HbA_{1c} levels and upper extremity problems in some studies, it is likely that poorer glycemic control over time with resulting AGE formation influences the development of hand and shoulder problems among patients with DM.

Calcific Shoulder Periarthritis (Tendinitis)

Calcific tendinitis is a painful condition most commonly affecting the shoulder in which calcium hydroxyapatite crystals deposit predominantly in periarticular areas. In the shoulder, these crystals may also deposit within the tendons of the rotator cuff. The incidence of calcific shoulder periarthritis is increased among patients with DM. In a case-control study, 824 hospitalized patients with type 2 diabetes and 320 age- and gender-matched hospitalized nondiabetic patients were evaluated with plain radiographs of the shoulder. Shoulder calcifications were evident in 31.8% of the patients with DM but in only 10% of controls without DM. Only 32.4% of those diabetics in whom calcific shoulder periarthritis had been diagnosed on plain radiographs experienced pain or limited range of motion.[62] Calcific tendonitis may coexist with adhesive capsulitis in the shoulder.

Carpal Tunnel Syndrome

Carpal tunnel syndrome (CTS) is an entrapment neuropathy caused by compression of the median nerve within the carpal tunnel. CTS presents with pain and paresthesias of the thumb, index, and middle fingers and of the radial aspect of the ring finger, which may be reproduced on physical examination by percussion of the median nerve at the wrist (Tinel's test) or on wrist dorsiflexion (Phalen's test). In diabetics, bilateral involvement of the median and ulnar nerves has been described, with resulting atrophy of the thenar, hypothenar, and intrinsic muscles of the hand and nerve conduction abnormalities.[63]

DM was identified as a risk factor of CTS in a large case-control study of 3391 patients who were identified as having CTS in the UK General Practice Research Database.[64] In another case-control study of 791 patients with CTS who were referred for electrodiagnostic studies, DM, female gender, obesity, and age between 41 and 60 years were observed significantly more frequently among patients with CTS. However, when these patients were stratified by body mass index (BMI), there no longer was a statistically significant association between DM and CTS, suggesting that obesity might have been a confounding factor. Although not a risk factor of unilateral CTS, DM is a risk factor of the development of bilateral CTS.[65] In a study of patients with type 1 or type 2 DM compared with control subjects without DM, Cagliero and colleagues[9] found that the prevalence of CTS among patients with DM was not significantly increased above that in nondiabetic controls.

The observation of simultaneous median and ulnar nerve involvement among patients with DM[63] and the doubled prevalence of CTS in the setting of diabetic polyneuropathy[66] raise the possibility that median neuropathy in diabetics may be caused by factors other than mechanical compression. The impaired median nerve regeneration and recovery observed after carpal tunnel release among some patients with DM suggests that intrinsic nerve pathology, in addition to external compression, might contribute to the pathogenesis of CTS in DM.[67–69] Proposed pathogenetic factors include hyperglycemia reducing myoinositol transport into nerves and increasing levels of endoneural free sugars, which may result in AGE modification of structural nerve proteins,[70] nerve ischemia causing endoneural hypoxia and demyelination,[71] and deficiencies of neurotrophic growth factors, such as nerve growth factor (NGF) and insulin-like growth factor (IGF)-1.[72] However, 2 subsequent prospective case-control studies found no difference in the rate of electrophysiologic recovery after carpal tunnel release when comparing patients with DM to nondiabetic controls or diabetic patients with polyneuropathy to those without.[73,74]

DIABETIC MUSCLE INFARCTION

DMI is an infrequent complication of DM that was first described in 1965 by Angervall as "tumoriform focal muscular degeneration."[75] Since its initial description, more than 100 cases have been reported.[76,77] More than half of these reported patients with DMI had type 1 DM with a mean duration of 15 years.

DMI almost always presents with the acute onset of muscle pain and swelling. The thigh muscles are most frequently involved in more than 80% of cases, but isolated calf muscle, simultaneous thigh and calf muscle, and upper extremity muscle involvement have been described. A palpable mass has been reported in 34% to 44% of cases. DMI recurred in the same or in a different muscle group in up to half the patients.

The mean mortality rate associated with DMI is 10% within 2 years of initial diagnosis; deaths occurred predominantly as a result of macrovascular complications.[78]

The diagnosis of DMI is based on a typical clinical presentation and characteristic findings on imaging studies. There is no specific laboratory marker for DMI. Serum creatine kinase (CK) levels were mentioned in fewer than half of the published cases and were elevated in slightly fewer than half of those patients for whom a level was reported. Typical findings on magnetic resonance imaging (MRI) include isointense swelling on T1-weighted images and diffuse heterogeneous hyperintensity on T2-weighted images of the affected muscle, with subcutaneous and subfascial edema. Gadolinium administration usually is not necessary, but nonenhancing areas surrounded by peripheral enhancement may be seen after contrast administration.[79] Muscle biopsy should be reserved for patients with an atypical clinical presentation, those in whom the diagnosis is uncertain, and those who do not improve with antiplatelet or anti-inflammatory drug therapy.[80] Histologic findings typically include muscle fiber necrosis, edema, phagocytosis of necrotic fibers, granulation tissue, and collagen deposition. Biopsy of more advanced lesions may reveal replacement of necrotic muscle fibers with fibrous tissue, regeneration of muscle fibers, and mononuclear infiltration of muscle.[76]

Because almost all reported patients with DMI have had microangiopathic complications of DM, such as retinopathy, nephropathy, or neuropathy, it has been suggested that reperfusion injury after muscle ischemia results in muscle infarction.[78] Hypercoagulability resulting from alteration of the coagulation-fibrinolytic system and endothelial dysfunction in DM have each been proposed as a potential pathogenic mechanism for the development of DMI.[81] Antiphospholipid antibodies have been hypothesized to contribute to the development of hypercoagulability in DM, but the number of patients with DMI and antiphospholipid antibodies has been insufficient to prove this association.[82]

Medical therapy with antiplatelet and/or anti-inflammatory drugs is recommended for DMI, but no randomized controlled trial has been performed because of the infrequent occurrence of this condition.[77]

NEUROPATHIC OSTEOARTHROPATHY (CHARCOT OSTEOARTHROPATHY, CHARCOT NEUROPATHIC ARTHROPATHY)

Neuropathic osteoarthropathy is a progressive, degenerative arthropathy associated with various diseases in which neuropathy occurs. In 1868, Charcot published a detailed description of this condition among patients with tabes dorsalis.[83] Subsequently, his name has been associated with the joint condition characterized by an inflammatory process that results in dislocation of the neuropathic joint and fracture and resorption of affected bones.

DM is the disease most commonly associated with neuropathic osteoarthropathy.[84] The prevalence of neuropathic osteoarthropathy among diabetics has been reported to be 0.15%. The joints most commonly involved include the true ankle, tarsometatarsal, metatarsophalangeal, and toe interphalangeal joints.[85]

Traditionally, neuropathic osteoarthropathy has been attributed to progressive joint and bone damage due to repeated weight-bearing trauma in the setting of decreased sensation caused by a sensory neuropathy (neurotraumatic theory). An alternative theory postulated that an autonomic neuropathy caused hyperemia, which resulted in stimulation of osteoclasts with increased bone resorption, osteoporosis, fractures, and joint damage (*neurovascular* theory).[86] Recently elucidated mechanisms of bone resorption suggest that increased expression of proinflammatory cytokines, such as TNF-α, may stimulate expression of the ligand for the receptor activator of nuclear factor κB (RANKL), which, by activating the nuclear transcription factor nuclear factor κB (NFκB), can induce the differentiation of precursor cells into osteoclasts that resorb bone. Normally, voluntary immobilization caused by pain limits this process. However, when pain sensation is impaired, the patient continues to walk and sustains repeated microtrauma that perpetuates inflammation and the resulting bone destruction.[87]

Because early immobilization is important to prevent progression of bone and joint damage, imaging studies should be obtained early in the course of disease, even if the patient is experiencing little pain. Initially, plain radiographs may demonstrate few abnormalities; however, bone marrow edema, bone bruising, or microfractures may be detected by MRI early in the course of neuropathic arthropathy.[88,89] Scintigraphic studies can differentiate neuropathic arthropathy from osteomyelitis. Combining indium-111-leukocyte (^{111}In-WBC) scanning with technetium-99 m-methylene diphosphonate (^{99}mTc-MDP) bone scanning virtually excludes osteomyelitis if both studies have negative results.[90–92]

DIFFUSE IDIOPATHIC SKELETAL HYPEROSTOSIS (FORESTIER'S DISEASE)

DISH is characterized by the calcification and ossification of ligaments and entheses. When first described in 1950 by Forestier and Rotes-Querol, it was called senile ankylosing hyperostosis of the spine. This name reflected its higher prevalence among older individuals, in contrast to ankylosing spondylitis, and its predilection for involving the axial skeleton, most often the thoracic spine.[93] Because this condition also can involve appendicular joints, the term *DISH* was introduced in 1976 by Resnick and Niwayama.[94]

In a cross-sectional study of 12,858 individuals older than 15 years, the prevalence of DISH was reported to be 3.5% among men and 2.2% among women older than 40 years.[95] The youngest patient diagnosed with DISH in that study was 43 years old.

DISH has been observed more often among patients with type 2 DM than in the general population, with an estimated prevalence of 13% to 40%.[96–98] However, other studies have found no significant increase in the prevalence of impaired glucose tolerance or DM in patients with DISH.[99–102] Among patients with DISH, the prevalence of metabolic syndrome is higher than among patients without DISH.[103,104]

Hyperinsulinemia has been suggested to link DM and obesity with the development of vertebral hyperostosis.[98,105] Insulin has been proposed as a factor that promotes bone growth in DISH.[106,107] In one study, patients with DISH and those with osteoarthritis (OA) had elevated levels of insulin and growth hormone (GH); however, levels of IGF-1 were higher in patients with DISH than in those with OA.[106] Both GH and IGF-1 may facilitate ossification of soft tissues in DISH by stimulating osteoblast proliferation and bone formation.[108]

The diagnosis of DISH is based on radiologic features. Radiographic criteria for the diagnosis of DISH proposed by Resnick and Niwayama in 1976 include the presence of "flowing" osteophytes along the anterolateral aspects of at least 4 contiguous vertebral bodies, the preservation of intervertebral disk spaces, and the absence of changes of degenerative spondylosis or spondyloarthropathy.[94] In 1985, Utsinger[109] proposed revised diagnostic criteria that incorporated involvement of peripheral entheses. He suggested that symmetric peripheral enthesopathy and continuous ossification along the anterolateral aspect of 2 or more contiguous vertebral bodies support a probable diagnosis of DISH.

Analgesics, heat application, exercise, and local corticosteroid injections have been used to treat patients with DISH but have not been studied in prospective, randomized, controlled clinical trials. In a 24-week study of a program of mobility, stretching, and strengthening exercises, 15 patients with DISH reported some improvement in spinal range of motion but no improvement in pain.[110]

CRYSTAL-INDUCED ARTHRITIS
Gout

In patients with gout, monosodium urate crystals are deposited in joints as a result of hyperuricemia. Acute attacks of gouty arthritis occur when intra-articular monosodium urate crystals are phagocytized by white blood cells that then release inflammatory mediators. The relationships between hyperuricemia, gout, and the metabolic syndrome have been evaluated in several cross-sectional studies. Epidemiologic studies have shown a higher prevalence of the metabolic syndrome among patients with hyperuricemia or gout. In a cross-sectional analysis of data obtained from 4053 young adults who participated in the Coronary Artery Risk Development in Young Adults (CARDIA) study, BMI, fasting insulin levels, and triglyceride levels were significantly higher among individuals with hyperuricemia.[111] Among 8669 participants in the Third National Health and Nutrition Examination Survey (NHANES III), the prevalence of the metabolic syndrome was greater with higher uric acid concentrations, ranging from 18.9% for individuals with serum uric acid levels of less than 6 mg/dL to 70.7% for those with serum uric acid levels of 10 mg/dL or greater.[112] In the same cohort, 62.8% of those with gout but only 25.4% of those without gout had the metabolic syndrome. After adjusting for age, gender, and known risk factors of development of the metabolic syndrome, such as BMI, hypertension, and DM, the likelihood of having the metabolic syndrome was found to be 3-fold greater if gout was present.[113]

Data from 2 epidemiologic studies also have demonstrated hyperuricemia to be a risk factor of the development of DM. In the Finnish Diabetes Prevention Study of 557 overweight and obese subjects with impaired glucose tolerance, hyperuricemia was established as a risk factor of DM after controlling for age, sex, hypertension, obesity, and hyperlipidemia.[114] In the Multiple Risk Factor Intervention Trial (MRFIT), a randomized, controlled trial designed to evaluate an interventional program for reducing the risk of developing coronary artery disease among men at high risk, hyperuricemia and gout were found to be risk factors of the development of type 2 DM. This association was established independent of age, BMI, smoking, family history of type 2 DM, diet, and presence of the metabolic syndrome and its individual components.[115]

The preponderance of patients with gout underexcrete uric acid through the kidney, which results in hyperuricemia; only a small proportion overproduce uric acid.[116] Thus, decreased renal uric acid excretion in the presence of hyperinsulinemia has been proposed as a potential link between hyperuricemia and both type 2 DM and the metabolic syndrome.[117-119] However, the association between hyperuricemia and gout, DM, and the metabolic syndrome remains an epidemiologic observation for which the molecular mechanism still needs to be elucidated.

Pseudogout

Calcium pyrophosphate dehydrate deposition in hyaline or fibrous cartilage, called chondrocalcinosis, may be asymptomatic. It often is identified as an incidental finding on plain radiographs. When symptomatic, it may manifest as acute or chronic inflammatory arthritis, called acute pseudogout or calcium pyrophosphate arthropathy, respectively. Although a relationship between pseudogout and DM has been suggested, there is a paucity of literature on this topic. The apparent association might be explained by the increased prevalence of both conditions among older individuals, with age being a confounding factor.[7,120–122] An association of pseudogout with DM has not been proven.

OSTEOARTHRITIS

Obesity is a known risk factor of the development of hip[123] and knee OA.[124–126] Despite the association of type 2 DM and the metabolic syndrome with obesity, there is no clinical evidence that DM or the metabolic syndrome predispose an individual to develop early or severe hip or knee OA.[127] However, there are features common to the pathogenesis of OA and of diabetic microvascular complications, such as AGEs and adipokinins.

In vitro, AGE modification increases the stiffness of normal articular cartilage,[128] reduces susceptibility of the cartilage to degradation by MMPs,[129] decreases proteoglycan synthesis by chondrocytes,[130,131] and increases chondrocyte-mediated proteoglycan degradation.[131] The observation that osteoarthritic cartilage is modified with AGEs has suggested a potential role for this process in the pathogenesis of OA. Adipokines, which are cytokines secreted by adipose tissue, may play a role in cartilage degeneration. Synovial fluid levels of the adipokine leptin are increased among patients with knee OA.[132] However, the mechanism by which leptin and other adipokines contribute to the pathogenesis of OA remains to be elucidated.

SUMMARY

DM is associated with various musculoskeletal manifestations. The strength of this relationship varies among the various musculoskeletal disorders; the associations are based mostly on epidemiologic data. For most of these conditions, definitive pathophysiologic correlates are lacking.

Hand and shoulder disorders occur more frequently than other musculoskeletal manifestations of DM. Recognition of the association between DM and shoulder adhesive capsulitis, DD, and stenosing flexor tenosynovitis facilitates their correct diagnosis in the setting of DM and prompt initiation of appropriate treatment, which may include optimizing glycemic control. Conversely, awareness and identification of the characteristic musculoskeletal manifestations of DM may facilitate earlier diagnosis of DM and initiation of glucose-lowering therapy to retard the development of diabetic complications.

Much less has been published about the musculoskeletal complications of DM than about its micro- and macrovascular complications. Prospective case-control cohort studies are needed to establish the true prevalence of musculoskeletal complications of DM and the metabolic syndrome, especially in this era of tighter glycemic control. The potential relationship between DM and the development of OA needs to be clarified in large, prospective, case-control cohort studies. The effect on musculoskeletal manifestations of various therapeutic regimens to manage DM should be studied prospectively. Treatment regimens for some musculoskeletal conditions associated with DM, such as DISH, should be studied in larger prospective, randomized, controlled clinical trials.

At the molecular level, further studies are warranted to clarify the potential contribution of AGEs and adipokines to the development of OA and diabetic musculoskeletal syndromes, such as shoulder adhesive capsulitis, DD, stenosing flexor tenosynovitis, and LJM. Identification of such molecular targets for therapy would promote the development of additional treatments for these and other rheumatic diseases.

REFERENCES

1. Cowie CC, Rust KF, Byrd-Holt DD, et al. Prevalence of diabetes and impaired fasting glucose in adults in the U.S. population: National Health And Nutrition Examination Survey 1999–2002. Diabetes Care 2006;29(6):1263–8.
2. American Diabetes Association. Diagnosis and classification of diabetes mellitus. Diabetes Care 2004;27(Suppl 1):S5–10.
3. Grundy SM, Cleeman JI, Daniels SR, et al. Diagnosis and management of the metabolic syndrome: an American Heart Association/National Heart, Lung, and Blood Institute scientific statement: Executive Summary. Crit Pathw Cardiol 2005;4(4):198–203.
4. Kahn R, Buse J, Ferrannini E, et al. The metabolic syndrome: time for a critical appraisal: joint statement from the American Diabetes Association and the European Association for the Study of Diabetes. Diabetes Care 2005;28(9): 2289–304.
5. Crispin JC, Alcocer-Varela J. Rheumatic manifestations of diabetes mellitus. Am J Med 2003;114:753–7.
6. Arkkila PE, Gautier JF. Musculoskeletal disorders in diabetes mellitus: an update. Best Pract Res Clin Rheumatol 2003;17(6):945–70.
7. Cagliero E. Rheumatic manifestations of diabetes mellitus. Curr Rheumatol Rep 2003;5(3):189–94.
8. Ardic F, Soyupek F, Kahraman Y, et al. The musculoskeletal complications seen in type II diabetics: predominance of hand involvement. Clin Rheumatol 2003; 22(3):229–33.
9. Cagliero E, Apruzzese W, Perlmutter GS, et al. Musculoskeletal disorders of the hand and shoulder in patients with diabetes mellitus. Am J Med 2002;112(6): 487–90.
10. Lundbaek K. Stiff hands in long-term diabetes. Acta Med Scand 1957;158: 447–51.
11. Rosenbloom AL, Frias JL. Diabetes mellitus, short stature and joint stiffness - a new syndrome. Clin Res 1974;22:92A.
12. Rosenbloom AL, Silverstein JH. Connective tissue and joint disease in diabetes mellitus. Endocrinol Metab Clin North Am 1996;25(2):473–83.
13. Rosenbloom AL. Limitation of finger joint mobility in diabetes mellitus. J Diabet Complications 1989;3(2):77–87.
14. Pal B, Anderson J, Dick WC, et al. Limitation of joint mobility and shoulder capsulitis in insulin- and non-insulin-dependent diabetes mellitus. Br J Rheumatol 1986;25(2):147–51.
15. Rosenbloom AL, Silverstein JH, Lezotte DC, et al. Limited joint mobility in childhood diabetes mellitus indicates increased risk for microvascular disease. N Engl J Med 1981;305(4):191–4.
16. Fitzcharles MA, Duby S, Waddell RW, et al. Limitation of joint mobility (cheiroarthropathy) in adult noninsulin-dependent diabetic patients. Ann Rheum Dis 1984;43(2):251–4.
17. Starkman HS, Gleason RE, Rand LI, et al. Limited joint mobility (LJM) of the hand in patients with diabetes mellitus: relation to chronic complications. Ann Rheum Dis 1986;45(2):130–5.

18. Arkkila PE, Kantola IM, Viikari JS, et al. Limited joint mobility is associated with the presence but does not predict the development of microvascular complications in type 1 diabetes. Diabet Med 1996;13(9):828–33.

19. Buckingham B, Perejda AJ, Sandborg C, et al. Skin, joint, and pulmonary changes in type I diabetes mellitus. Am J Dis Child 1986;140(5):420–3.

20. Lawson PM, Maneschi F, Kohner EM. The relationship of hand abnormalities to diabetes and diabetic retinopathy. Diabetes Care 1983;6(2):140–3.

21. Jennings AM, Milner PC, Ward JD. Hand abnormalities are associated with the complications of diabetes in type 2 diabetes. Diabet Med 1989;6(1):43–7.

22. Arkkila PE, Kantola IM, Viikari JS. Limited joint mobility in type 1 diabetic patients: correlation to other diabetic complications. J Intern Med 1994; 236(2):215–23.

23. Arkkila PE, Kantola IM, Viikari JS, et al. Shoulder capsulitis in type I and II diabetic patients: association with diabetic complications and related diseases. Ann Rheum Dis 1996;55(12):907–14.

24. McCance DR, Crowe G, Quinn MJ, et al. Incidence of microvascular complications in type 1 diabetic subjects with limited joint mobility: a 10-year prospective study. Diabet Med 1993;10(9):807–10.

25. Arkkila PE, Kantola IM, Viikari JS. Limited joint mobility in non-insulin-dependent diabetic (NIDDM) patients: correlation to control of diabetes, atherosclerotic vascular disease, and other diabetic complications. J Diabetes Complications 1997;11(4):208–17.

26. Vukovic J, Dumic M, Radica A, et al. Risk factors for expression and progression of limited joint mobility in insulin-dependent childhood diabetes. Acta Diabetol 1996;33(1):15–8.

27. Silverstein JH, Gordon G, Pollock BH, et al. Long-term glycemic control influences the onset of limited joint mobility in type 1 diabetes. J Pediatr 1998; 132(6):944–7.

28. Aydeniz A, Gursoy S, Guney E. Which musculoskeletal complications are most frequently seen in type 2 diabetes mellitus? J Int Med Res 2008;36(3): 505–11.

29. Lindsay JR, Kennedy L, Atkinson AB, et al. Reduced prevalence of limited joint mobility in type 1 diabetes in a U.K. clinic population over a 20-year period. Diabetes Care 2005;28(3):658–61.

30. Harris MI, Klein R, Welborn TA, et al. Onset of NIDDM occurs at least 4–7 yr before clinical diagnosis. Diabetes Care 1992;15(7):815–9.

31. Infante JR, Rosenbloom AL, Silverstein JH, et al. Changes in frequency and severity of limited joint mobility in children with type 1 diabetes mellitus between 1976–78 and 1998. J Pediatr 2001;138(1):33–7.

32. Eaton RP, Sibbitt WL Jr, Harsh A. The effect of an aldose reductase inhibiting agent on limited joint mobility in diabetic patients. JAMA 1985;253(10):1437–40.

33. Krans HM. Recent clinical experience with aldose reductase inhibitors. J Diabetes Complications 1992;6(1):39–44.

34. Kameyama M, Meguro S, Funae O, et al. The presence of limited joint mobility is significantly associated with multiple digit involvement by stenosing flexor tenosynovitis in diabetics. J Rheumatol 2009;36(8):1686–90.

35. Yosipovitch G, Yosipovitch Z, Karp M, et al. Trigger finger in young patients with insulin dependent diabetes. J Rheumatol 1990;17(7):951–2.

36. Chammas M, Bousquet P, Renard E, et al. Dupuytren's disease, carpal tunnel syndrome, trigger finger, and diabetes mellitus. J Hand Surg Am 1995;20(1): 109–14.

37. Ryzewicz M, Wolf JM. Trigger digits: principles, management, and complications. J Hand Surg Am 2006;31(1):135–46.
38. Baumgarten KM, Gerlach D, Boyer MI. Corticosteroid injection in diabetic patients with trigger finger. A prospective, randomized, controlled double-blinded study. J Bone Joint Surg Am 2007;89(12):2604–11.
39. Wang AA, Hutchinson DT. The effect of corticosteroid injection for trigger finger on blood glucose level in diabetic patients. J Hand Surg Am 2006;31(6):979–81.
40. Griggs SM, Weiss AP, Lane LB, et al. Treatment of trigger finger in patients with diabetes mellitus. J Hand Surg Am 1995;20(5):787–9.
41. Stahl S, Kanter Y, Karnielli E. Outcome of trigger finger treatment in diabetes. J Diabetes Complications 1997;11(5):287–90.
42. Noble J, Heathcote JG, Cohen H. Diabetes mellitus in the aetiology of Dupuytren's disease. J Bone Joint Surg Br 1984;66(3):322–5.
43. Loos B, Puschkin V, Horch RE. 50 years experience with Dupuytren's contracture in the Erlangen University Hospital–a retrospective analysis of 2919 operated hands from 1956 to 2006. BMC Musculoskelet Disord 2007;8:60.
44. Arkkila PE, Kantola IM, Viikari JS, et al. Dupuytren's disease in type 1 diabetic patients: a five-year prospective study. Clin Exp Rheumatol 1996;14(1):59–65.
45. Hurst LC, Badalamente MA, Hentz VR, et al. Injectable collagenase clostridium histolyticum for Dupuytren's contracture. N Engl J Med 2009;361(10):968–79.
46. Reeves B. The natural history of the frozen shoulder syndrome. Scand J Rheumatol 1975;4(4):193–6.
47. Codman EA. Tendinitis of the short rotators. In: Codman EA, editor. The shoulder: rupture of the supraspinatus tendon and other lesions in or about the subacromial bursa. Boston: Thomas Todd Co; 1934. p. 216–24. Chapter VII.
48. Neviaser J. Adhesive capsulitis of the shoulder. J Bone Joint Surg Am 1945;27:211–22.
49. Bridgman JF. Periarthritis of the shoulder and diabetes mellitus. Ann Rheum Dis 1972;31(1):69–71.
50. Balci N, Balci MK, Tuzuner S. Shoulder adhesive capsulitis and shoulder range of motion in type II diabetes mellitus: association with diabetic complications. J Diabetes Complications 1999;13(3):135–40.
51. Ramchurn N, Mashamba C, Leitch E, et al. Upper limb musculoskeletal abnormalities and poor metabolic control in diabetes. Eur J Intern Med 2009;20(7):718–21.
52. Bunker TD, Anthony PP. The pathology of frozen shoulder. A Dupuytren-like disease. J Bone Joint Surg Br 1995;77(5):677–83.
53. Bunker TD, Reilly J, Baird KS, et al. Expression of growth factors, cytokines and matrix metalloproteinases in frozen shoulder. J Bone Joint Surg Br 2000;82(5):768–73.
54. Griggs SM, Ahn A, Green A. Idiopathic adhesive capsulitis. A prospective functional outcome study of nonoperative treatment. J Bone Joint Surg Am 2000;82-A(10):1398–407.
55. Ogilvie-Harris DJ, Myerthall S. The diabetic frozen shoulder: arthroscopic release. Arthroscopy 1997;13(1):1–8.
56. Cinar M, Akpinar S, Derincek A, et al. Comparison of arthroscopic capsular release in diabetic and idiopathic frozen shoulder patients. Arch Orthop Trauma Surg 2010;130(3):401–6.
57. Sheridan MA, Hannafin JA. Upper extremity: emphasis on frozen shoulder. Orthop Clin North Am 2006;37(4):531–9.
58. Buckingham BA, Uitto J, Sandborg C, et al. Scleroderma-like changes in insulin-dependent diabetes mellitus: clinical and biochemical studies. Diabetes Care 1984;7(2):163–9.

59. Yamagishi S, Imaizumi T. Diabetic vascular complications: pathophysiology, biochemical basis and potential therapeutic strategy. Curr Pharm Des 2005; 11(18):2279–99.
60. Yamagishi S. Advanced glycation end products and receptor-oxidative stress system in diabetic vascular complications. Ther Apher Dial 2009;13(6):534–9.
61. Monnier VM, Vishwanath V, Frank KE, et al. Relation between complications of type I diabetes mellitus and collagen-linked fluorescence. N Engl J Med 1986;314(7):403–8.
62. Mavrikakis ME, Drimis S, Kontoyannis DA, et al. Calcific shoulder periarthritis (tendinitis) in adult onset diabetes mellitus: a controlled study. Ann Rheum Dis 1989;48(3):211–4.
63. Jung Y, Hohmann TC, Gerneth JA, et al. Diabetic hand syndrome. Metabolism 1971;20(11):1008–15.
64. Geoghegan JM, Clark DI, Bainbridge LC, et al. Risk factors in carpal tunnel syndrome. J Hand Surg Br 2004;29(4):315–20.
65. Becker J, Nora DB, Gomes I, et al. An evaluation of gender, obesity, age and diabetes mellitus as risk factors for carpal tunnel syndrome. Clin Neurophysiol 2002;113(9):1429–34.
66. Perkins BA, Olaleye D, Bril V. Carpal tunnel syndrome in patients with diabetic polyneuropathy. Diabetes Care 2002;25(3):565–9.
67. Ozkul Y, Sabuncu T, Kocabey Y, et al. Outcomes of carpal tunnel release in diabetic and non-diabetic patients. Acta Neurol Scand 2002;106(3):168–72.
68. Yasuda H, Terada M, Maeda K, et al. Diabetic neuropathy and nerve regeneration. Prog Neurobiol 2003;69(4):229–85.
69. Kennedy JM, Zochodne DW. Impaired peripheral nerve regeneration in diabetes mellitus. J Peripher Nerv Syst 2005;10(2):144–57.
70. Greene DA, Lattimer SA, Sima AA. Sorbitol, phosphoinositides, and sodium-potassium-ATPase in the pathogenesis of diabetic complications. N Engl J Med 1987;316(10):599–606.
71. Low PA, Tuck RR, Dyck PJ, et al. Prevention of some electrophysiologic and biochemical abnormalities with oxygen supplementation in experimental diabetic neuropathy. Proc Natl Acad Sci U S A 1984;81(21):6894–8.
72. Chiarelli F, Santilli F, Mohn A. Role of growth factors in the development of diabetic complications. Horm Res 2000;53(2):53–67.
73. Thomsen NO, Cederlund R, Rosen I, et al. Clinical outcomes of surgical release among diabetic patients with carpal tunnel syndrome: prospective follow-up with matched controls. J Hand Surg Am 2009;34(7):1177–87.
74. Mondelli M, Padua L, Reale F, et al. Outcome of surgical release among diabetics with carpal tunnel syndrome. Arch Phys Med Rehabil 2004; 85(1):7–13.
75. Angervall L, Stener B. Tumoriform focal muscular degeneration in two diabetic patients. Diabetologia 1965;1:39–42.
76. Trujillo-Santos AJ. Diabetic muscle infarction: an underdiagnosed complication of long-standing diabetes. Diabetes Care 2003;26(1):211–5.
77. Kapur S, McKendry RJ. Treatment and outcomes of diabetic muscle infarction. J Clin Rheumatol 2005;11(1):8–12.
78. Kapur S, Brunet JA, McKendry RJ. Diabetic muscle infarction: case report and review. J Rheumatol 2004;31(1):190–4.
79. Kattapuram TM, Suri R, Rosol MS, et al. Idiopathic and diabetic skeletal muscle necrosis: evaluation by magnetic resonance imaging. Skeletal Radiol 2005; 34(4):203–9.

80. Chester CS, Banker BQ. Focal infarction of muscle in diabetics. Diabetes Care 1986;9(6):623–30.
81. Bjornskov EK, Carry MR, Katz FH, et al. Diabetic muscle infarction: a new perspective on pathogenesis and management. Neuromuscul Disord 1995; 5(1):39–45.
82. Palmer GW, Greco TP. Diabetic thigh muscle infarction in association with anti-phospholipid antibodies. Semin Arthritis Rheum 2001;30(4):272–80.
83. Charcot J. Sur quelques arthropathies qui paraissent dependre d'une lesion du cerveau ou de la moelle epiniere. Arch Physiol Norm Pathol 1868;1:161–78.
84. Lee L, Blume PA, Sumpio B. Charcot joint disease in diabetes mellitus. Ann Vasc Surg 2003;17(5):571–80.
85. Sinha S, Munichoodappa CS, Kozak GP. Neuro-arthropathy (Charcot joints) in diabetes mellitus (clinical study of 101 cases). Medicine (Baltimore) 1972; 51(3):191–210.
86. Brower AC, Allman RM. Pathogenesis of the neurotrophic joint: neurotraumatic vs. neurovascular. Radiology 1981;139(2):349–54.
87. Jeffcoate WJ. Charcot neuro-osteoarthropathy. Diabetes Metab Res Rev 2008; 24(Suppl 1):S62–5.
88. Chantelau E, Richter A, Ghassem-Zadeh N, et al. "Silent" bone stress injuries in the feet of diabetic patients with polyneuropathy: a report on 12 cases. Arch Orthop Trauma Surg 2007;127(3):171–7.
89. Ulbrecht JS, Wukich DK. The Charcot foot: medical and surgical therapy. Curr Diab Rep 2008;8(6):444–51.
90. Lipman BT, Collier BD, Carrera GF, et al. Detection of osteomyelitis in the neuropathic foot: nuclear medicine, MRI and conventional radiography. Clin Nucl Med 1998;23(2):77–82.
91. Palestro CJ, Mehta HH, Patel M, et al. Marrow versus infection in the Charcot joint: indium-111 leukocyte and technetium-99m sulfur colloid scintigraphy. J Nucl Med 1998;39(2):346–50.
92. Seabold JE, Flickinger FW, Kao SC, et al. Indium-111-leukocyte/technetium-99 m-MDP bone and magnetic resonance imaging: difficulty of diagnosing osteomyelitis in patients with neuropathic osteoarthropathy. J Nucl Med 1990;31(5): 549–56.
93. Forestier J, Rotes-Querol J. Senile ankylosing hyperostosis of the spine. Ann Rheum Dis 1950;9(4):321–30.
94. Resnick D, Niwayama G. Radiographic and pathologic features of spinal involvement in diffuse idiopathic skeletal hyperostosis (DISH). Radiology 1976;119(3):559–68.
95. Julkunen H, Heinonen OP, Pyorala K. Hyperostosis of the spine in an adult population. Its relation to hyperglycaemia and obesity. Ann Rheum Dis 1971;30(6): 605–12.
96. Julkunen H, Karava R, Viljanen V. Hyperostosis of the spine in diabetes mellitus and acromegaly. Diabetologia 1966;2(2):123–6.
97. Hajkova Z, Streda A, Skrha F. Hyperostotic spondylosis and diabetes mellitus. Ann Rheum Dis 1965;24(6):536–43.
98. Kiss C, Szilagyi M, Paksy A, et al. Risk factors for diffuse idiopathic skeletal hyperostosis: a case-control study. Rheumatology (Oxford) 2002;41(1): 27–30.
99. Mader R, Dubenski N, Lavi I. Morbidity and mortality of hospitalized patients with diffuse idiopathic skeletal hyperostosis. Rheumatol Int 2005; 26(2):132–6.

100. Mata S, Fortin PR, Fitzcharles MA, et al. A controlled study of diffuse idiopathic skeletal hyperostosis. Clinical features and functional status. Medicine (Baltimore) 1997;76(2):104–17.
101. Sencan D, Elden H, Nacitarhan V, et al. The prevalence of diffuse idiopathic skeletal hyperostosis in patients with diabetes mellitus. Rheumatol Int 2005; 25(7):518–21.
102. Daragon A, Mejjad O, Czernichow P, et al. Vertebral hyperostosis and diabetes mellitus: a case-control study. Ann Rheum Dis 1995;54(5):375–8.
103. Vezyroglou G, Mitropoulos A, Antoniadis C. A metabolic syndrome in diffuse idiopathic skeletal hyperostosis. A controlled study. J Rheumatol 1996;23(4): 672–6.
104. Mader R, Novofestovski I, Adawi M, et al. Metabolic syndrome and cardiovascular risk in patients with diffuse idiopathic skeletal hyperostosis. Semin Arthritis Rheum 2009;38(5):361–5.
105. Littlejohn GO, Smythe HA. Marked hyperinsulinemia after glucose challenge in patients with diffuse idiopathic skeletal hyperostosis. J Rheumatol 1981;8(6): 965–8.
106. Denko CW, Boja B, Moskowitz RW. Growth promoting peptides in osteoarthritis and diffuse idiopathic skeletal hyperostosis–insulin, insulin-like growth factor-I, growth hormone. J Rheumatol 1994;21(9):1725–30.
107. Littlejohn GO. Insulin and new bone formation in diffuse idiopathic skeletal hyperostosis. Clin Rheumatol 1985;4(3):294–300.
108. Ernst M, Rodan GA. Increased activity of insulin-like growth factor (IGF) in osteoblastic cells in the presence of growth hormone (GH): positive correlation with the presence of the GH-induced IGF-binding protein BP-3. Endocrinology 1990; 127(2):807–14.
109. Utsinger PD. Diffuse idiopathic skeletal hyperostosis. Clin Rheum Dis 1985; 11(2):325–51.
110. Al-Herz A, Snip JP, Clark B, et al. Exercise therapy for patients with diffuse idiopathic skeletal hyperostosis. Clin Rheumatol 2008;27(2):207–10.
111. Rathmann W, Funkhouser E, Dyer AR, et al. Relations of hyperuricemia with the various components of the insulin resistance syndrome in young black and white adults: the CARDIA study. Coronary Artery Risk Development in Young Adults. Ann Epidemiol 1998;8(4):250–61.
112. Choi HK, Ford ES. Prevalence of the metabolic syndrome in individuals with hyperuricemia. Am J Med 2007;120(5):442–7.
113. Choi HK, Ford ES, Li C, et al. Prevalence of the metabolic syndrome in patients with gout: the Third National Health and Nutrition Examination Survey. Arthritis Rheum 2007;57(1):109–15.
114. Niskanen L, Laaksonen DE, Lindstrom J, et al. Serum uric acid as a harbinger of metabolic outcome in subjects with impaired glucose tolerance: the Finnish Diabetes Prevention Study. Diabetes Care 2006;29(3):709–11.
115. Choi HK, De Vera MA, Krishnan E. Gout and the risk of type 2 diabetes among men with a high cardiovascular risk profile. Rheumatology (Oxford) 2008;47(10): 1567–70.
116. Boss GR, Seegmiller JE. Hyperuricemia and gout: classification, complications and management. N Engl J Med 1979;300:1459–68.
117. Facchini F, Chen YD, Hollenbeck CB, et al. Relationship between resistance to insulin-mediated glucose uptake, urinary uric acid clearance, and plasma uric acid concentration. JAMA 1991;266(21):3008–11.

118. Ter Maaten JC, Voorburg A, Heine RJ, et al. Renal handling of urate and sodium during acute physiological hyperinsulinaemia in healthy subjects. Clin Sci (Lond) 1997;92(1):51–8.
119. Muscelli E, Natali A, Bianchi S, et al. Effect of insulin on renal sodium and uric acid handling in essential hypertension. Am J Hypertens 1996;9(8):746–52.
120. McCarty DJ, Silcox DC, Coe F, et al. Diseases associated with calcium pyrophosphate dihydrate crystal deposition. Am J Med 1974;56(5):704–14.
121. Alexander GM, Dieppe PA, Doherty M, et al. Pyrophosphate arthropathy: a study of metabolic associations and laboratory data. Ann Rheum Dis 1982;41(4): 377–81.
122. Jones AC, Chuck AJ, Arie EA, et al. Diseases associated with calcium pyrophosphate deposition disease. Semin Arthritis Rheum 1992;22(3):188–202.
123. Cooper C, Inskip H, Croft P, et al. Individual risk factors for hip osteoarthritis: obesity, hip injury, and physical activity. Am J Epidemiol 1998;147(6):516–22.
124. Felson DT, Anderson JJ, Naimark A, et al. Obesity and knee osteoarthritis. The Framingham Study. Ann Intern Med 1988;109(1):18–24.
125. Cooper C, Snow S, McAlindon TE, et al. Risk factors for the incidence and progression of radiographic knee osteoarthritis. Arthritis Rheum 2000;43(5): 995–1000.
126. Niu J, Zhang YQ, Torner J, et al. Is obesity a risk factor for progressive radiographic knee osteoarthritis? Arthritis Rheum 2009;61(3):329–35.
127. Burner TW, Rosenthal AK. Diabetes and rheumatic diseases. Curr Opin Rheumatol 2009;21(1):50–4.
128. Verzijl N, DeGroot J, Ben ZC, et al. Crosslinking by advanced glycation end products increases the stiffness of the collagen network in human articular cartilage: a possible mechanism through which age is a risk factor for osteoarthritis. Arthritis Rheum 2002;46(1):114–23.
129. DeGroot J, Verzijl N, Wenting-Van Wijk MJ, et al. Age-related decrease in susceptibility of human articular cartilage to matrix metalloproteinase-mediated degradation: the role of advanced glycation end products. Arthritis Rheum 2001;44(11):2562–71.
130. DeGroot J, Verzijl N, Bank RA, et al. Age-related decrease in proteoglycan synthesis of human articular chondrocytes: the role of nonenzymatic glycation. Arthritis Rheum 1999;42(5):1003–9.
131. DeGroot J, Verzijl N, Jacobs KM, et al. Accumulation of advanced glycation endproducts reduces chondrocyte-mediated extracellular matrix turnover in human articular cartilage. Osteoarthritis Cartilage 2001;9(8):720–6.
132. Gandhi R, Takahashi M, Syed K, et al. Relationship between body habitus and joint leptin levels in a knee osteoarthritis population. J Orthop Res 2010;28(3): 329–33.

Adrenal Disorders in Rheumatology

Michelle J. Ormseth, MD[a],*, John S. Sergent, MD[b]

KEYWORDS

• Adrenal • Cushing syndrome
• Hypothalamic pituitary adrenal axis • Glucocorticoid
• Rheumatologic • Autoimmune

Knowledge of both adrenal insufficiency and Cushing syndrome are important in the care of patients with rheumatologic disease due to clinical similarities in relation to glucocorticoid in rheumatologic diseases. Difficulties in differentiating between adrenal insufficiency and active or worsening disease often arise when glucocorticoids are tapered in patients with conditions such as vasculitis and polymyositis. In addition there are striking similarities with adrenal insufficiency and diseases such as fibromyalgia syndrome and polymyalgia rheumatica. Similarly, the proximal muscle symptoms of Cushing syndrome can be mistaken for several other disorders such as polymyositis. Osteoporosis is a major concern in patients with endogenous and glucocorticoid-induced Cushing syndrome.

ADRENAL INSUFFICIENCY
Definition

Adrenal insufficiency is classified into three subtypes based on where the abnormality is based in the hypothalamic pituitary adrenal (HPA) axis. Primary insufficiency is caused by adrenal gland damage. The secondary form is related to insufficient corticotrophin (ACTH) from the pituitary gland. The tertiary form is related to insufficient corticotrophin-releasing hormone (CRH) from the hypothalamus.

Acute adrenal insufficiency, or adrenal crisis, is severe and characterized by shock. This is often related to mineralocorticoid deficiency, but not always in severe cases related to exogenous glucocorticoid withdrawal. Chronic primary adrenal insufficiency

The authors have nothing to disclose.

[a] Division of Rheumatology and Immunology, Department of Medicine, Vanderbilt University Medical Center, Vanderbilt University School of Medicine, 1161 21st Avenue South, T-3219 MCN, Nashville, TN 37232-2681, USA

[b] Department of Internal Medicine, Vanderbilt University Medical Center, 1161 21st Avenue South, D-3100 MCN, Nashville, TN 37232-2358, USA

* Corresponding author.
E-mail address: Michelle.ormseth@vanderbilt.edu

Rheum Dis Clin N Am 36 (2010) 701–712
doi:10.1016/j.rdc.2010.09.005
0889-857X/10/$ – see front matter © 2010 Elsevier Inc. All rights reserved.

is related to deficiency of glucocorticoid, mineralocorticoid, and even androgen deficiency in women.

Causes and Associations with Rheumatologic Disease

Primary adrenal insufficiency, or Addison disease, initially was most commonly related to tuberculosis, but now is typically caused by autoimmune adrenalitis in the Western world (69% to 91.2%).[1,2] Additionally, in one retrospective study, a concomitant autoimmune disorder was seen in nearly 50% of patients with autoimmune adrenalitis, including most commonly autoimmune thyroid disease and vitiligo, but less commonly Sjogren syndrome.[1] Although concomitant connective tissue disease is only occasionally reported in literature (in addition to Sjogren syndrome), there are also reports of systemic lupus erythematosis,[3] rheumatoid arthritis,[4] systemic sclerosis,[5,6] Takayasu arteritis, and ankylosing spondylitis.[7] More frequently thrombosis of the adrenal gland, caused by antiphospholipid antibody syndrome, is seen.[8–12] Polyglandular autoimmune syndrome type II (APSII) has some reported association with rheumatoid arthritis[13] and Sjogren syndrome.[14] The reported association with rheumatologic disease is infrequent and may be coincidence; association with polyglandular autoimmune syndrome type I is not reported. This may be because of differences in HLA type.[15]

Secondary adrenal insufficiency can be related to the destruction of the pituitary gland or deficiency of ACTH. Classically, this is associated with hemorrhage of the pituitary gland, or thrombosis such as seen when sarcoidosis affects the pituitary gland.[16] There have been a few reports of opiate induced secondary adrenal insufficiency.[17,18] Glucocorticoid use can cause secondary or tertiary adrenal insufficiency.

Tertiary adrenal insufficiency is most commonly related to withdrawal of glucocorticoids. Glucocorticoid-induced adrenal insufficiency can be caused by several mechanisms, including decreased hypothalamic synthesis of CRH, blockade of the actions of CRH on the anterior pituitary, and, after prolonged or profound deficiency of ACTH, adrenal atrophy.[19,20]

Adrenal crisis can occur in patients with all forms of adrenal insufficiency, but more often is associated with primary adrenal insufficiency. The trigger can be infection or other major stress with no or insufficient glucocorticoid intake. Certainly, bilateral adrenal hemorrhage or infarction and pituitary infarction can cause this also. Abrupt discontinuation of corticosteroids and inadequate supplementation in stress are other causes of adrenal crisis.

Signs and Symptoms

The symptoms of adrenal crisis are more severe than chronic adrenal insufficiency. The distinguishing feature of adrenal crisis is shock, and other signs and symptoms depend on whether the patient has underlying primary or secondary adrenal insufficiency. **Table 1** displays the signs and symptoms of adrenal insufficiency.

Chronic adrenal insufficiency is more difficult to diagnose, as presenting symptoms can be vague. A recent comprehensive review of cases of hypoadrenalism reported in literature since its characterization over 150 years ago showed that the most common symptoms of adrenal insufficiency are arthralgias, myalgias, back pain, and decreased joint movement. Those with primary adrenal insufficiency additionally frequently had fatigue, gastrointestinal symptoms, hyperpigmentation, weight loss, hypotension, and postural dizziness.[21] Painful lower extremity flexion contractures of the muscles of the pelvic girdle, hips, and knees are common signs in autoimmune primary adrenal insufficiency and pituitary causes are often seen with isolated deficiency of ACTH.[22–24]

Table 1
Similarities between adrenal insufficiency and fibromyalgia syndrome

	Primary	Secondary/ Glucocorticoid- Induced	Fibromyalgia
Symptoms			
Myalgia	xxx	xxx	xxx
Arthralgia	xxx	xxx	xxx
Back pain	xxx	xx	x
Fatigue	xxx	xxx	xxx
Gastrointestinal symptoms[a]	xx	x	x
Postural dizziness	x	x	x
Hypogonadism		xx[b]	
Psychiatric	x	x	xxx
Poor sleep			xxx
Signs			
Hyperpigmentation	xx		
Weight loss	xx	x	
Flexion contracture	x[c]	xx[c]	
Hypotension	xx	x	
Hyponatremia	xx	x	
Hyperkalemia	xx	x	
Hypoglycemia		x	
Anemia	xx	x	

[a] Gastrointestinal symptoms include nausea, vomiting, diarrhea.
[b] In the setting of hypopituitarism.
[c] In general associated with autoimmune and pituitary causes.

Rheumatology Mimickers and Methods of Differentiation

Adrenal insufficiency can look much like fibromyalgia syndrome. **Table 1** compares various forms of adrenal insufficiency and fibromyalgia syndrome. Widespread pain with emphasis on muscles and joints is most common complaint in fibromyalgia patients.[25] In addition to more commonly recognized symptoms of pain, stiffness, fatigue, sleep disturbance, and mood disorder of fibromyalgia syndrome,[26] patients can have disabling dizziness.[27] The important differentiating factors for these diseases are the physical signs of disease such as electrolyte abnormalities, flexion contractures, and hypotension; however, these are not always present in adrenal insufficiency.

Polymyalgia rheumatica (PMR) can look quite similar to adrenal insufficiency. With stiffness, pain, malaise, weight loss, and fever, the best differentiating factor is the elevated acute phase reactants in polymyalgia rheumatica.

When considering the differential diagnosis of arthralgia and myalgia it is important to recall that adrenal insufficiency is the only one characterized by predominant lower limb pain.[21] This difference may be helpful when proposing an appropriate initial workup.

Glucocorticoid-induced Adrenal Insufficiency

A major concern to physicians is glucocorticoid-induced adrenal insufficiency caused by HPA axis suppression. In the course of steroid taper, a patient may develop steroid withdrawal syndrome or true adrenal insufficiency. The symptomatology is very similar, but the withdrawal syndrome displays normal HPA axis testing, and these patients do not develop adrenal crisis.[28] The symptoms can develop despite supraphysiologic steroid dose.[29] The underlying cause of the withdrawal syndrome may be related to elevated interleukin (IL)-6.[30]

The symptoms of glucocorticoid-induced adrenal insufficiency are listed in **Table 1**, but it can notably manifest as adrenal crisis. It can occur in the setting of medical and surgical stress and also with concomitant use of certain medications, whether it be through increased steroid metabolism with rifampicin or decreased absorption with bile acid sequestrants. **Table 2** shows several culprit medications.

Dose, duration of use, and potency of the glucocorticoid factor into the risk of HPA axis suppression. However, even inhaled corticosteroids, if abruptly withdrawn, can promote adrenal insufficiency.[31] If possible to do, alternate-day dosing of oral glucocorticoids may be helpful to prevent suppression of the HPA axis.[32]

There have been no prospective studies to determine the best method of steroid taper. Although it has not been tested in randomized placebo-controlled trial, the authors recommend when tapering high-dose glucocorticoids that at the point when taper can be initiated, gradually taper prednisone equivalent to 5 mg over 6 months then decrease by 1 mg per month.

Diagnosis of Adrenal Insufficiency

There are several tests involved in the evaluation of adrenal insufficiency. Baseline morning (6–8 am) cortisol level less than 83 nmol/L or less than 3 μg/dL is diagnostic of adrenal insufficiency, whereas levels greater than 550 nmol/L or 20 μg/dL at anytime exclude it.[33] If initial evaluation does not provide a diagnosis, the short 250 μg ACTH (cosyntropin) stimulation test may be performed; after baseline cortisol level is obtained, 250 μg ACTH is administered, and cortisol is measured 30 to 60 minutes later. If the adrenal gland cannot produce the normal 18 μg/dL or 500 nmol or greater response, it is indicative of primary adrenal insufficiency or other forms after functional adrenal gland atrophy occurs.[34] This test can be normal in central adrenal insufficiency, however. The insulin-induced hypoglycemia test can be helpful to determine if the patient has a deficiency in ACTH, but can be dangerous given the induction of hypoglycemia in particularly the elderly and those with cardiovascular disease. Thus, the CRH stimulation test can be used alternatively, but it can be costly. An overnight metyrapone test can help to diagnose secondary adrenal insufficiency caused by disruption of cortisol synthesis, but obtaining the drug can be difficult. Finally,

Table 2
Medications that change the metabolism or availability of glucocorticoids

Decrease GC Levels	Increase GC Levels
Barbiturates[80]	Antiretrovirals, especially ritonavir[81]
Bile acid sequestrants[82]	Azole antifungals, fluconazole
Mitotane[83]	Clarithromycin[84]
Primidone[85]	Estrogen derivatives
Rifampicin[86–88]	Itraconazole[89]
Somatropin[90]	Macrolides except for azithromycin and spiramycin
	Nondihydropyridine calcium channel blockers

Abbreviation: GC, glucocorticoid.

the low-dose ACTH stimulation can be performed, but it may not supply much more information compared with the high-dose test.[35]

Special considerations are necessary if the patient is taking glucocorticoids. Given the limited half-life of the drugs, testing can be performed before administration of daily morning glucocorticoid dose. In general, if there is difficulty tapering the glucocorticoid dose below physiologic levels because of symptoms suggestive of adrenal insufficiency, evaluation via the 250 µg ACTH stimulation test may be helpful, and, if necessary, the CRH stimulation test may be used to confirm.[36]

HPA Axis Dysfunction in Rheumatologic Disease

There has been the suggestion that inadequate HPA axis response to a stress and chronic exposure to the stressor may be contributing factors to autoimmune disease.[37] Rheumatoid arthritis patients have inappropriately low cortisol levels for their inflammatory status and have low adrenal androgens.[38,39] Similarly, HPA axis abnormalities have been shown in Sjogren syndrome and systemic lupus erythematosus,[40,41] and seem to promote chronic inflammation.[42] There are low dehydroepiandrosterone (DHEA) and DHEA sulfate (DHEAS) levels in Sjogren syndrome patients, and DHEA supplementation was shown to slightly improve symptoms of dry mouth in one study.[43]

Low serum DHEA levels are common in systemic lupus erythematosus, and low levels correlate with active disease.[44] Studies looking at supplementation of DHEA are conflicting. A 6-month open-label study looking at lupus patients with mild-to-moderate disease showed significant reduction in Systemic Lupus Erythematosus Activity Index (SLEDAI) (from 10.0 ± 2.9 to 4.9 ± 1.7, $P = .04$) and a decrease in daily corticosteroid requirement.[45] However, a 3-month double-blind randomized placebo-controlled trial of patients with mild-to-moderate lupus showed no statistically significant difference in the SLEDAI or corticosteroid use.[46] Another randomized, double-blind placebo-controlled trial of patients with active lupus showed that supplementation with DHEA 200 mg/d resulted in a sustained reduction of prednisone dose in 51% in the treatment group versus 29% in the placebo group ($P = .031$).[47] The same conflicting information is present in looking at the benefit to fatigue and well-being.[48,49]

PMR, as mentioned, has major presenting symptomatic similarities to adrenal insufficiency as well as resolution of symptoms with administration of glucocorticoids. It has been asserted that PMR is an HPA-axis driven disease.[50] Given inflammatory status, patients with PMR have low serum cortisol levels on or off corticosteroids.[51] A study evaluating the HPA axis in PMR patients showed that these patients have lower cortisol and adrenal androgen, DHEAS, and this was related to abnormal adrenal response to ACTH stimulation.[52]

CUSHING SYNDROME
Definition and Causes

Cushing syndrome is a term given to a collection of manifestations caused by hypercortisolism. The most common cause is exogenous glucocorticoid administration. Endogenous Cushing syndrome is far less common. Causes include Cushing disease, an overproduction of ACTH caused by pituitary adenoma, ectopic ACTH production, or overproduction of cortisol in the adrenal glands. Under-recognized sources of Cushing syndrome include inhaled[53] and topical preparations,[54] intra-articular joint injections,[55] and even Chinese herbal medicines, which may contain various types of glucocorticoids.[56] **Table 2** shows several medications that can increase exogenous glucocorticoid levels, increasing the risk of Cushing syndrome.

Signs and Symptoms

The signs and symptoms of Cushing syndrome include

Central obesity with moon face and buffalo hump
Thin skin
Large purple striae
Cataracts
Poor wound healing
Lower extremity edema
Spontaneous tendon rupture, muscle wasting, particularly in the lower proximal limbs
Osteoporosis
Insulin resistance
Hypertension and cardiovascular disease
Arterial and venous thrombosis
Psychiatric disturbance
Hirsutism
Gonadal dysfunction (related to adrenocortical androgens).[57–60]

Polyarthropathy can develop in Cushing syndrome, but it most likely related to avascular necrosis of multiple joints, which is more common in glucocorticoid-associated than spontaneous Cushing syndrome.[61,62] Endogenous Cushing syndrome can mask or induce remission in steroid-responsive disease such as rheumatoid arthritis.[63,64] Some patients with Cushing disease can have cyclical episodes of active hypercortisolism or just have one predominant feature.[65] This can cause delays and confusion in diagnosis.

Interestingly, while patients with endogenous Cushing syndrome have increased cardiovascular disease, the use of glucocorticoids does not appear to be associated with increased risk of cardiovascular disease, at least in patients with polymyalgia rheumatica, rheumatoid arthritis, and systemic lupus erythematosus.[66–68]

Dose, duration of use, and potency of the glucocorticoid factor into the risk of glucocorticoid-induced myopathy. Short-term high-dose corticosteroid use results in acute diffuse myopathy, atrophy, and even rhabdomyolysis.[69] Chronic use results in chronic myopathy manifested with proximal muscle weakness. The equivalent of 10 mg prednisone daily is an unusual cause of myopathy, but doses of 40 to 60 mg/d can cause weakness within 2 weeks.[70] Fluorinated glucocorticoid preparations are more often associated with myopathy than nonfluorinated glucocorticoid preparations.[71]

Osteoporosis

Osteoporosis is a considerable threat in Cushing syndrome. Even subclinical Cushing syndrome can result in osteoporosis.[72] The relative risk of low-energy fractures in patients with endogenous Cushing syndrome was 5.4 compared with controls, but there was a sharp decline in risk after treatment.[73] Despite that sharp decline, the duration of subsequent glucocorticoid replacement is a stronger predictor of low bone density than the duration of untreated Cushing syndrome.[74]

Not only does glucocorticoid use, particularly high-dose glucocorticoid use, cause rapid loss of trabecular bone mineral density, but it also causes loss of lean body mass, which together increase the risk of fracture.[75] This bone loss is rapid in the first 6 months of treatment, declining by approximately 5% in the first year, but subsequent loss is 1% to 2% per year.[76] In one study, this translated into 17% of patients developing a vertebral fracture in the first year of glucocorticoid use.[77] While alternate-day

Table 3
Differential diagnosis of proximal muscle symptoms and method of differentiation

	Creatine Kinase	Pain	Weakness
Cushing syndrome	nl/sl↑	-	+
Polymyositis/Dermatomyositis	↑	-	+
Polymyalgia rheumatica	nl	+	-
Hypothyroidism[91]	↑	+	+
Vitamin D deficiency[92]	nl	+	±
Fibromyalgia syndrome	nl	+	-
Statin myopathy	↑	+	+
Myasthia gravis	nl	-	+
Muscular dystrophy	↑	-	+

dosing possibly may help prevent adrenal insufficiency, it does not help prevent bone loss.[78]

Rheumatology Mimickers and Methods of Differentiation

Important to the differential diagnosis of proximal muscle weakness are Cushing syndrome, both endogenous and glucocorticoid-induced, and inflammatory myopathy such as polymyositis. **Table 3** shows a comparison of disorders causing proximal muscle symptoms. In particular, differentiating between active polymyositis and glucocorticoid-induced myopathy in a patient with known polymyositis can be very difficult. Tapering the glucocorticoid dose and monitoring serial urinary creatine may be helpful, as this will decrease with the discontinuation of steroids in the setting of glucocorticoid-induced myopathy as opposed to increasing with polymyositis.[79]

Diagnosis of Cushing Syndrome

After exclusion of exogenous glucocorticoid use, the recommendation from the Endocrine Society is to evaluate the patient with a high diagnostic accuracy test. If this is abnormal, the patient should be referred to endocrinologist for further evaluation.[58] The initial tests include late night salivary cortisol (at least two measurements), urinary free cortisol (at least two measurements), and a low-dose dexamethasone suppression test.

SUMMARY

Understanding adrenal disorders, whether endogenous or related to glucocorticoid use is important to the day-to-day care of patients with rheumatologic disease.

REFERENCES

1. Zelissen PM, Bast EJ, Croughs RJ. Associated autoimmunity in Addison's disease. J Autoimmun 1995;8(1):121–30.
2. Kasperlik-Zaluska AA, Migdalska B, Czarnock B, et al. Association of Addison's disease with autoimmune disorders—a long-term observation of 180 patients. Postgrad Med J 1991;67(793):984–7.
3. Lenaerts J, Vanneste S, Knockaert D, et al. SLE and acute Addisonian crisis due to bilateral adrenal hemorrhage: association with the antiphospholipid syndrome. J Tenn Med Assoc 1996;89:120.

4. Robinson C. Addison's disease and rheumatoid arthritis. Ann Rheum Dis 1957; 16:82–3.
5. Saba G, Pallone E, Micheli G. Case of primary adrenocortical insufficency associated with scleroderma. G Clin Med 1969;50:369–77.
6. Koskova E, Rovensky J, Simorova E, et al. Systemic scleroderma and Addison's disease. Isr Med Assoc J 2005;7:130–1.
7. Zhang Z, Wang Y, Zhou W, et al. Addison's disease secondary to connective tissue disease: a report of six cases. Rheumatol Int 2009;29:647–50.
8. Takebayashi K, Aso Y, Tayama K, et al. Primary antiphospholipid syndrome associated with acute adrenal failure. Am J Med Sci 2003;325:441–4.
9. Asherson RA, Hughes GR. Recurrent deep vein thrombosis and Addison's disease in "primary" antiphospholipid syndrome. J Rheumatol 1989;16:378–80.
10. Gonzalez G, Gutierrex M, Ortiz M, et al. Association of primary antiphospholipid syndrome with primary adrenal insufficiency. J Rheumatol 1996;23:1286–7.
11. Satta M, Corsello S, Casa S, et al. Adrenal insufficiency as the first clinical manifestation of the primary antiphospholipid antibody syndrome. Horumon To Rinsho 2000;52:123–6.
12. Espinosa G, Cervera R, Font J, et al. Adrenal involvement in the antiphospholipid syndrome. Lupus 2003;12:569–72.
13. Cicchinelli M, Mariani M, Scuderi F. Polyglandular autoimmune syndrome type II and rheumatoid arthritis. Clin Exp Rheumatol 1997;15:336–7.
14. Ergas D, Tsimanis A, Shtalrid M, et al. T-gamma large granular lymphocyte leukemia associated with amegakaryocytic thrombocytopenic purpura, Sjogren's syndrome, and polyglandular autoimmune syndrome type II, with subsequent development of pure red cell aplasia. Am J Hematol 2002;69:132–4.
15. Wallaschofski H, Meyer A, Tuschy U, et al. HLA-DQA1*0301-associated susceptibility for autoimmune polyglandular syndrome type II and III. Horm Metab Res 2003;35:120–4.
16. Gostiljac D, Dordevic P, Maric-zivkovic J, et al. Sarcoidosis localized in endocrine glands. Med Pregl 2005;58:25–9.
17. Mussig K, Knaus-Dittmann D, Schmidt H, et al. Secondary adrenal failure and secondary amenorrhoea following hydromorphone treatment. Clin Endocrinol (Oxf) 2007;66:604.
18. Schimke K, Greminger P, Brandle M. Secondary adrenal insufficiency due to opiate therapy – another differential diagnosis worth consideration. Exp Clin Endocrinol Diabetes 2009;117:649–51.
19. Jasani M, Boyle J, Greig W, et al. Corticosteroid-induced suppression of the hypothalamo-pituitary-adrenal axis: observations on patients given oral corticosteroids for rheumatoid arthritis. QJM 1967;36:261–76.
20. Krasner A. Glucocorticoid-induced adrenal insufficiency. JAMA 1999;282:671–6.
21. Sathi N, Makkuni D, Mitchell W, et al. Musculoskeletal aspects of hypoadrenalism: just a load of aches and pains? Clin Rheumatol 2009;28:631–8.
22. Berger J, Herregods P, Verhelst J, et al. Flexion contractures in secondary adrenal insufficiency. Clin Rheumatol 2010;29:115–7.
23. Odagaki T, Noguchi Y, Fukui T. Flexion contractures of the legs as the initial manifestation of adrenocortical insufficiency. Intern Med 2003;42:710–3.
24. Syriou V, Moisidis A, Tamouridis N, et al. Isolated adrenocorticotropin deficiency and flexion contractures syndrome. Hormones (Athens) 2008;7:320–4.
25. Hauser W, Zimmer C, Felde E, et al. What are the key symptoms of fibromyalgia. Results of a survey of the German Fibromyalgia Association. Schmerz 2008;22: 176–83.

26. Boomershine C, Crofford L. A symptom-based approach to pharmacologic management of fibromyalgia. Nat Rev Rheumatol 2009;5:191–9.

27. Staud R. Autonomic dysfunction in fibromyalgia syndrome: postural orthostatic tachycardia. Curr Rheumatol Rep 2008;10:463–6.

28. Amatruda T, Hollingsworth D, D'Esopo N, et al. A study of the mechanism of the steroid withdrawal syndrome: evidence for integrity of the hypothalamic-pituitary-adrenal-system. J Clin Endocrinol Metab 1960;20:339–54.

29. Dixon R, Christy N. On the various forms of corticosteroid withdrawal syndrome. Am J Med 1980;68:224–30.

30. Papanicolaou D, Tsigos C, Oldfield E, et al. Acute glucorticoid deficiency is associated with plasma elevations in interleukin-6: does that latter participate in the symptomatology of the steroid withdrawal syndrome and adrenal insufficiency? J Clin Endocrinol Metab 1996;81:2303–6.

31. Molimard M, Girodet P, Pollet C, et al. Inhaled corticosteroids and adrenal insufficiency: prevalence and clinical presentation. Drug Saf 2008;31:769–74.

32. Axelrod L. Glucocorticoid therapy. Medicine 1976;55:39–65.

33. May M, Carey R. Rapid adrenocorticotropic hormone test in practice. Retrospective review. Am J Med 1985;79:679–84.

34. Dickstein G, Shechner C, Nicholson W, et al. Adrenocorticotropin stimulation test: effects of basal cortisol level, time of day, and suggested new sensitive low dose test. J Clin Endocrinol Metab 1991;72:773–8.

35. Mayenknecht J, Diedrich S, Bahr V, et al. Comparison of low and high dose corticotropin stimulation tests in patients with pituitary disease. J Clin Endocrinol Metab 1998;83:1558–62.

36. Schlaghecke R, Kornely E, Santen R, et al. The effect of long-term glucocorticoid therapy on pituitary adrenal responses to exogenous corticotrophin releasing hormone. N Engl J Med 1992;326:226–30.

37. Cutolo M, Prete C, Walker J. Is stress a factor in the pathogenesis in autoimmune rheumatic diseases? Clin Exp Rheumatol 1999;17:515–8.

38. Straub R, Paimela L, Peltomaa R, et al. Inadequately low serum levels of steroid hormones in relation to IL-6 and TNF in untreated patients with early rheumatoid arthritis and reactive arthritis. Arthritis Rheum 2002;46:654–62.

39. Bulsma J, Cutolo M, Masi A, et al. Neuroendocrine immune basis of the rheumatic diseases. Immunol Today 1999;20:298–301.

40. Johnson E, Vlachoyiannopoulos P, Skopouli F, et al. Hypofunction of the stress axis in Sjogren's syndrome. J Rheumatol 1998;25:1508–14.

41. Zietz B, Reber T, Oertel M, et al. Altered function of the hypothalamic stress axis in patients with moderately active systemic lupus erythematosus. II. Dissociation between androstenedione, cortsol, or dehydroepiandrosterone and interleukin 6 or tumor necrosis factor. J Rheumatol 2000;27:911–8.

42. Dillon J. Dehydroepiandrosterone, dehydroepiandrosterone sulfate and related steroids: theis role in inflammatory, allergic and immunological disorders. Curr Drug Targets Inflamm Allergy 2005;4:377–85.

43. Forsblad-d'Elia H, Carlsten H, Labrie F, et al. Low serum levels of sex steroids are associated with disease characteristics in primary Sjogren's syndrome; supplementation with dehydroepiandrosterone restores the concentrations. J Clin Endocrinol Metab 2009;94(6):2044–51.

44. Lahita R, Bradlow H, Ginzler E, et al. Low plasma androgens in women with systemic lupus erythematosus. Arthritis Rheum 1987;30:241–8.

45. vanVollenhoven R, Engleman E, McGuire J. An open study of dehydroepiandrosterone in systemic lupus erythematosus. Arthritis Rheum 1994;37:1305–10.

46. vanVollenhoven R, Engleman E, McGuire J. Dehydroepiandrosterone in systemic lupus erythematosus. Results of a double-blind, placebo-controlled, randomized clinical trial. Arthritis Rheum 1995;38:1826–31.

47. Petri M, Lahita R, vanVollenhoven R, et al. Effects of prasterone on corticosteroid requirements of women with systemic lupus erythematosus: a double-blind, randomized, placebo-controlled trial. Arthritis Rheum 2002;46:1820–9.

48. Nordmark G, Bengtsson C, Larsson A, et al. Effects of dehydroepiandrosterone supplementation on health-related quality of life in glucocorticoid treated female patients with systemic lupus erythematosus. Autoimmunity 2005;38:531–40.

49. Hartkamp A, Greenen R, Godaert G, et al. Effects of dehydrepiandrosterone on fatigue and well-being in women with quiescent systemic lupus erythematosus: a randomized controlled trial. Ann Rheum Dis 2010;69:1144–7.

50. Cutolo M, Straub R. Polymyalgia rheumatica: evidence for a hypothalamic-pituitary adrenal axis-driven disease. Clin Exp Rheumatol 2000;18:655–8.

51. Staub R, Gluck T, Cutolo M, et al. The adrenal steroid status in relation to inflammatory cytokines (interleukin-6 and tumor necrosis factor) in polymyalgia rheumatica. Rheumatology 2000;39:624–31.

52. Cutolo M, Salvarani C, Sulli A, et al. Adrenal gland hypofunction in early-onset polymyalgia rheumatica. Effects of 12 months of corticosteroid treatment on adrenal hormones and IL-6 levels. J Rheumatol 2002;29:748–56.

53. Chalkley S, Chisholm D. Cushing's syndrome from an inhaled glucocorticoid. Med J Aust 1994;160:611, 614–5.

54. Walsh P, Aeling J, Huff L, et al. Hypothalamus-pituitary-adrenal axis suppression by superpotent topical steroids. J Am Acad Dermatol 1993;29:501.

55. Gondwe J, Davidson J, Deeley S, et al. Cushing's syndrome in children with juvenile idiopathic arthritis following intra-articular triamcinolone acetonide administration. Rheumatology (Oxford) 2005;44:1457–8.

56. Edwards C, Lian T, Chng H. Cushing's syndrome caused by treatment of gout with traditional Chinese medicine. QJM 2002;95:705.

57. Newell-Price J, Bertagna X, Grossman A, et al. Cushings syndrome. Lancet 2006; 367:1605–17.

58. Nieman L, Biller B, Findling J, et al. The diagnosis of Cushings's syndrome: an endocrine society clinical practice guideline. J Clin Endocrinol Metab 2008;93:1526–40.

59. Findling J, Raff H. Cushing's syndrome: important issues in diagnosis and management. J Clin Endocrinol Metab 2006;91:3746–53.

60. Kelly W, Kelly M, Faragher B. A prospective study of psychiatric and psychological aspects of Cushing's syndrome. Clin Endocrinol (Oxf) 1996;45:715–20.

61. Kingsley G, Hickling P. Polyarthropathy associated with Cushing's disease. Br Med J (Clin Res Ed) 1986;292:1363.

62. Wicks I, Calligeros D, Kidson W, et al. Cushing's disease presenting with avascular necrosis of the femoral heads and complicated by pituitary apoplexy. Ann Rheum Dis 1987;46:783–6.

63. Uthman I, Senecal J. Onset of rheumatoid arthritis after surgical treatment of Cushing's disease. J Rheumatol 1995;22:1964–6.

64. Yakushiji F, Kita M, Hiroi N, et al. Exacerbation of rheumatoid arthritis after removal of adrenal adenoma in Cushing's Syndrome. Endocr J 1995;42:219–23.

65. Bertagna X, Guignat L, Groussin L, et al. Cushing's disease. Best Pract Res Clin Endocrinol Metab 2009;23:607–23.

66. Kremers H, Reinalda M, Crowson C, et al. Glucocorticoids and cardiovascular and cerebrovascular events in polymyalgia rheumatica. Arthritis Rheum 2007; 57:279–86.

67. Nurmohamed M, van Halm V, Dijkmans B. Cardiovascular risk profile of antirheumatic agents in patients with osteoarthritis and rheumatoid arthritis. Drugs 2002; 62:1599–609.
68. Bruce I. 'Not only...but also': factors that contribute to accelerated atherosclerosis and premature coronary heart disease in systemic lupus erythematosus. Rheumatology (Oxford) 2005;44:1492–502.
69. Williams T, O'Hehir R, Czarny D, et al. Acute myopathy in severe acute asthma treated with intravenously administered corticosteroids. Am Rev Respir Dis 1988;137:460–3.
70. Bowyer S, LaMothe M, Hollister J. Steroid myopathy: incidence and detection in a population with asthma. J Allergy Clin Immunol 1985;76:234–42.
71. Anagnos A, Ruffi R, Kaminiski H. Endocrine myopathies. Neurol Clin 1997;15: 673–96.
72. Sippel R, Chen H. Subclinical Cushing's syndrome in adrenal incidentalomas. Surg Clin North Am 2004;84:875–85.
73. Vastergaard P, Lindholm J, Jorgensen J, et al. Increased risk of osteoporotic fractures in patients with Cushing's syndrome. Eur J Endocrinol 2002;146:51–6.
74. Barahona M, Sucunza N, Resmini E, et al. Deleterious effects of glucocorticoid replacement on bone in women after long-term remission of Cushing's syndrome. J Bone Miner Res 2009;24:1841–6.
75. Natsui K, Tanaka K, Suda M, et al. High-dose glucocorticoid treatment induces rapid loss of trabecular bone mineral density and lean body mass. Osteoporos Int 2006;17:105–8.
76. Baxter JD. Advances in glucocorticoid therapy. Adv Intern Med 2000;45:317–49.
77. Cohen S, Levy R, Keller M, et al. Risedronate therapy prevents corticosteroid-induced bone loss: a twelve-month, multicenter, randomized, double-blind, placebo-controlled, parallel-group study. Arthritis Rheum 1999;42:2309–18.
78. Ruegsegger P, Medici T, Anliker M. Corticosteroid-induced bone loss. A longitudinal study of alternate day therapy in patients with bronchial asthma using quantitative computed tomography. Eur J Clin Pharmacol 1983;25:615–20.
79. Askari A, Vignos P, Moskowitz R. Steroid myopathy in connective tissue disease. Am J Med 1976;61:485–92.
80. Putignano P, Kaltsas G, Satta M, et al. The effects of anti-convulsant drugs on adrenal function. Horm Metab Res 1998;30:389–97.
81. Pessanha T, Campos J, Barros A, et al. Iatrogenic Cushing's syndrome in a adolescent with AIDs on ritonavir and inhaled fluticasone. Case report and literature review. AIDS 2007;21:529–32.
82. Gambertoglio J, Amend W, Benet L. Pharmacokinetic and bioavailability of prednisone and prednisolone in healthy volunteers and patients: a review. J Pharmacokinet Biopharm 1980;8:1–52.
83. Robinson B, Hales I, Henniker A, et al. The effect of o, p′-DDD on adrenal steroid replacement therapy requirements. Clin Endocrinol (Oxf) 1987;27:437–44.
84. DeWachter E, Malfroot A, DeSchutter I, et al. Inhaled budesonide induced Cushings's syndrome in cystic fibrosis patients, due to drug inhibition of cytochrome P450. J Cyst Fibros 2003;2:72–5.
85. Patsalos P, Duncan J. Antiepileptic drugs. A review of clinically significant drug interactions. Drug Saf 1993;9:156–84.
86. Okudaira S, Shimoji K, Yogi Y, et al. A case of partial Addison's disease activated with the administration of rifampicin (RFP). Kekkaku 1999;74(2):115–20.
87. Kyriazopoulou V, Parparousi O, Vagenakis A. Rifampicin-induced adrenal crisis in addisonian patients receiving corticosteroid replacement therapy. J Clin Endocrinol Metab 1984;59:1204–6.

88. San Jose A, Simo R, Cierco P, et al. Adrenal insufficiency crisis after treatment with rifampicin. Med Clin (Barc) 1987;89:397.

89. DeWachter E, Vanbesien J, DeSchutter I, et al. Rapidly developing Cushing syndrome in a 4-year-old patient during combined treatment with itraconazole and inhaled budesonide. Eur J Pediatr 2003;162:488–9.

90. Scaroni C, Ceccato F, Rizzati S, et al. Concomitant therapies (glucocorticoids and sex hormones) in adult patients with growth hormone deficiency. J Endocrinol Invest 2008;31:61–5.

91. Hekimsoy Z, Oktem I. Serum creatine kinase levels in overt and subclinical hypothyroidism. Endocr Res 2005;31:171–5.

92. Al-Said Y, Al-Rached H, Al-Qahtani H, et al. Severe proximal myopathy with remarkable recovers after vitamin D treatment. Can J Neurol Sci 2009;36:336–9.

Arthropathy in Acromegaly

Z. Killinger, MD, PhD[a], J. Payer, MD, PhD[a], I. Lazúrová, MD, PhD[b],
R. Imrich, MD, PhD[c], Z. Homérová, MD[a], M. Kužma, MD[a],
J. Rovenský, MD, DSc, FRCP[d,e],*

KEYWORDS

- Arthropathy in acromegaly • Definition
- Epidemiology and pathogenesis
- Musculoskeletal manifestation • Treatment of acromegaly

DEFINITION

Acromegaly is a chronic and slowly developing endocrinopathy caused by hypersecretion of growth hormone (GH) and consequently of insulinlike growth factor 1 (IGF-1) due to GH-secreting pituitary tumor. Other causes, such as increased growth hormone–releasing hormone production from hypothalamic tumors, ectopic growth hormone–releasing hormone production, and ectopic GH secretion from nonendocrine tumors, are rare.

EPIDEMIOLOGY AND PATHOGENESIS

Acromegaly most commonly occurs in middle-aged men and women. Its prevalence is approximately 4.6 cases per million population, and the incidence is 116.9 new cases per million per year.[1]

Hypersecretion of GH affects all organs, causing disturbances in morphology, endocrine function, and metabolism. GH released into circulation stimulates production of IGF-1, which is the primary mediator of the growth-promoting effects of GH. GH stimulates growth of soft tissue and fibroblast proliferation too, causing an increased thickening of connective tissue. GH also has other actions that are not mediated by IGF-I, such as anti-insulin, lipolytic, and natriuretic effects. There are also local manifestations presented by growth of pituitary adenoma, which may compress local structures and cause neurologic symptomatology.[2]

[a] Fifth Internal Clinic, University Hospital, Ružinovská 6, 826 06 Bratislava, Slovakia
[b] First Department of Internal Medicine, Medical Faculty, Trieda SNP 1, 040 00 Košice, Slovakia
[c] Center for Molecular Medicine, Institute of Experimental Endocrinology, Slovak Academy of Science, Vlárska 3, 831 01 Bratislava, Slovakia
[d] National Institute of Rheumatic Diseases, Nábrezie Ivana Krasku 4, 921 12 Piešťany, Slovakia
[e] SS. Cyril and Methodius University in Trnava, Institute the Physiotherapy, Balneology and Therapeutic Rehabilitation, Rázusova s. 14, 921 01 Piešťany, Slovakia
* Corresponding author. National Institute of Rheumatic Diseases, 921 12 Piešťany, Slovakia.
E-mail address: rovensky.jozef@nurch.sk

Rheum Dis Clin N Am 36 (2010) 713–720
doi:10.1016/j.rdc.2010.09.004
0889-857X/10/$ – see front matter

CLINICAL FEATURES OF ACROMEGALY

The most typical features of acromegaly are listed in **Box 1**.[3]

PROGNOSIS

Prognosis of acromegaly is dependent on early detection and treatment of the disease. Acromegalic patients demonstrate a 2- to 4-fold increase in mortality relative to the general population.

MUSCULOSKELETAL MANIFESTATIONS

Musculoskeletal pain is a frequent problem encountered in acromegaly and is associated with a reduction in quality of life. Joint symptoms are the most frequent complaint, affecting approximately 70% of individuals at the time of diagnosis. Among musculoskeletal symptoms, the most prevalent are arthropathy, carpal tunnel syndrome, proximal myopathy, and fibromyalgia. A less discussed but frequent sign is bone mass alteration leading to osteoporosis.

Acromegalic Arthropathy

The articular manifestations of acromegaly are one of the most frequent clinical complications and may be present as the earliest symptom in a significant proportion of patients. Their prevalence and severity worsen with the duration of uncontrolled disease and often result in significant disability.

Arthropathy in acromegaly has been recognized since Pierre Marie's classical description of the disease in 1886.[4]

The pathogenesis of arthropathy in acromegaly is comprised of two mechanisms: initial endocrine and subsequent mechanical changes. First, in the early course of the disease, elevated GH and IGF-I levels promote growth of the articular cartilage and periarticular ligaments, which leads to cartilage thickening and joint space congestion. These changes cause limitation in the range of movements, and overgrown ligaments cause laxity of the joint.

Radiologic changes in this early phase are joint space widening and periarticular soft tissue hypertrophy (**Fig. 1**). This first mechanism is likely to occur early in the course of the disease and is at least partially reversible with adequate disease control. With ongoing disease, arthropathy becomes irreversible and biochemical control of acromegaly, as documented by a normal IGF-I, will have small efficacy in improving the clinical status. Altered joint geometry results in repeated intra-articular trauma and exaggerated reparative reactions, which leads to scar, cysts, and osteophyte formation with further worsening of joint geometry. At this point, the disease acquires the characteristics and features of degenerative joint disease.[5] Radiographic changes at this stage are characterized by narrowing of joint spaces, osteophytosis, cysts, and other features typical for the later stages of the disease (see **Box 2**).[6]

The radiologic appearance of arthropathy in acromegaly was mostly studied in small noncontrolled groups of patients with untreated or treated but active disease. These studies have suggested that more severe radiologic abnormalities were related to biochemically more active acromegaly and longer disease duration.[6]

Clinical features of arthropathy in acromegaly

Arthralgia is one of the most common complaints of acromegalic patients (up to 75% of patients).[3] Sixty percent to 70% of patients have involvement of large peripheral joints (shoulder, knee, and hip). Back pain may be a particularly troubling feature of acromegaly. Approximately 50% of patients have axial arthropathy affecting mainly the lumbar area. Patients complain of dull diffuse pain in the lumbar region. The pain does not radiate into the legs and is often present both in rest and in activity.[7]

Further common complaints relate to limited range of movement, joint instability, and joint deformation. The presence of radiologic abnormalities and clinical manifestations of arthropathy are not correlated, unless joints are severely affected, as in long-standing disease.[5]

A recent study evaluated 89 acromegalic patients with adequate long-term disease control for prevalence and radiologic characteristics of arthropathy. They found evidence for radiologic arthritis in a least one joint in all patients and clinical arthritis in two-thirds of patients. The most prevalent manifestation was axial osteoarthritis, affecting the cervical and lumbar areas, even at young ages. The characteristic radiologic changes observed were wide joint spaces and severe osteophytosis.[6]

In the early phase of the disease, widened intervertebral spaces and vertebral enlargement may be present on a spine radiograph.

Ossification of the anterior surface of vertebral bodies is common and in more severe cases can bridge the disc space, resembling diffuse idiopathic skeletal hyperostosis syndrome.

Biermasz and colleagues[1] reported that a high prevalence of self-reported joint complaints persisted despite successful long-term treatment of acromegaly. These joint problems were an important indicator of impaired quality of life.[8]

Carpal Tunnel Syndrome

CTS occurs in approximately 30% to 50% of acromegalic patients and is frequently bilateral. Compression and hypertrophy of the median nerve are the most important factors in the pathogenesis of the syndrome. In a Spanish study, musculoskeletal involvement was the second most frequent cause of morbidity in acromegaly with the prevalence of CTS up to 19%.[9] In the study of Miller and colleagues,[10] 17.2% of 58 acromegalic patients had previously undergone carpal tunnel decompression and 39.7% had symptoms of CTS at diagnosis. Moreover, subclinical CTS was even more common, reaching a prevalence of 81%. It is presumable that the incidence of CTS reflects the greater sensitivity of the inching method for detecting focal conduction abnormalities. Several studies documented that improvement of CTS symptoms occurs with decreased GH secretion after surgery or radiotherapy for acromegaly. In the study of Kameyama after adenomectomy or radiotherapy, nerve conduction normalized in 26% patients.[11] In addition, surgical reports documented that besides causal treatment of GH overproduction, open carpal tunnel release for median nerve decompression should prove an effective treatment for CTS in acromegaly.[12]

Bone Mass Alterations and Fracture Risk in Acromegaly

Although acromegaly is often included in lists of endocrinopathies associated with osteoporosis due to increased bone turnover, some investigators have reported normal or increased bone mass in this disorder.[13]

During childhood, GH secretion stimulates linear bone growth via its effect on IGF-I. The effects of GH secretion due to acromegaly on skeletal mass and bone metabolism in adults have been somewhat conflicting.

GH and IGF-I have a stimulatory effect on osteoblast function and several studies indicate a potential anabolic effect of GH, at least on the cortical bone. Acromegalics had significantly higher levels of osteocalcin than controls. Seeman and colleagues

Box 1
Clinical features of acromegaly

General effects
- Soft tissue swelling
- Acral enlargement

Musculoskeletal/neurologic effects
- Arthralgia
- Prognathism
- Arthropathy
- Paraesthesia
- Carpal tunnel syndrome

Local tumor effects
- Visual impairment
- Headaches
- Pituitary infarction
- Cranial nerve impingement

Cutaneous effects
- Cosmetic disfigurement
- Increased sweating
- Acne
- Greasy skin
- Skin tags

Gastrointestinal effects
- Colonic polyps, carcinoma
- Enlarged organ size

Cardiovascular and respiratory effects
- Hypertension
- Cardiac enlargement

Fatigue
- Tongue enlargement
- Sleep apnea syndrome
- Daytime somnolence
- Voice changes

Endocrine and metabolic changes
- Carbohydrate intolerance
- Diabetes mellitus
- Hyperphosphatemia/Hypercalciuria
- Hyperlipidemia
- Goiter
- Hyperprolactinemia

Psychosexual effects

 Decreased libido

 Menstrual disturbances

 Impotence

 Depression/decreased vitality

Data from Harris AG. Acromegaly and its management. Philadelphia: Lippincott-Raven; 1996. p. 24–35.

demonstrated that osteoporosis occurs rarely in acromegaly. If present, it could be a consequence of hypogonadism. Characteristically, acromegaly causes an increase both in bone apposition and resorption; data on bone mass are controversial. This discordance of results depends mainly on differences in skeletal sites investigated, diagnostic equipment used and grouping of patients regardless of gender and gonadal status. Data on cortical bone generally show a normal or even increased

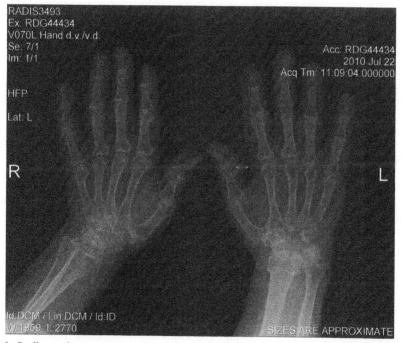

Fig. 1. Radiograph comparing views of hands, dorsovolar projection, of a 72-year-old woman with diagnosis of acromegaly. At the joint margins of distal and proximal interphalangeal joints and carpal joints are visualized osteophytic apositions more significant on the right hand. Metacarpal boneheads of the right hand are enlarged by rounded exostotic formations; articular spaces of metacarpophalangeal joints are widened bilaterally. Fine periosteal reactions of medial and proximal phalangs at the filamented compact bone are more transparent. Increased transparency of bones on the right hand declares the presence of diffuse osteoporosis. Radiograph view of acromegaly is more probable at the view marked as right hand (R). (*Courtesy of* Peter Vaňuga, PhD. National Institute of Endocrinology and Diabetology. Lubochňa, Slovakia.)

Box 2
Radiologic findings in acromegalic joint disease

Increased joint space diameter

Decreased joint space diameter (severe disease)

Tufting of distal phalanges

Enthesopathy

Angular joint deformities

Osteophyte formation

Articular surface calcification

Eburnation

Subchondral cyst formation

Costochondral joint calcification and enlargement

Vertebral body enlargement

Data from Harris AG. Acromegaly and its management. Philadelphia: Lippincott-Raven; 1996. p. 24–35; with permission.

---

bone mineral density (regardless of the gonadal status), whereas discrepant data are available on the trabecular bone.[3]

Some of the inconsistencies in the literature can be accounted for by the common association of acromegaly and hypogonadism. The impact of hypogonadism should, therefore, be considered in patients with acromegaly when evaluating bone density.

In some studies, an increased propensity to fracture has not been reported in acromegalic patients. Alternatively, a small cross-sectional study of 36 postmenopausal acromegalic women showed that those with active disease had higher vertebral bone mineral density but also a higher prevalence of vertebral fractures compared with inactive acromegalics patients. The overall risk of fracture was not increased among acromegalics compared with normal controls.[14] In 2005, Bonnadonna and colleagues[15] pointed to a high prevalence of radiologic vertebral fractures in postmenopausal women with active acromegaly. Osteoporotic vertebral fractures are also often asymptomatic and underdiagnosed in these patients.[16]

TREATMENT OF ACROMEGALY

Surgery is indicated when there is a large tumor with impingement of the optic chiasm or nerve and in all other cases of a high presurgical likelihood of complete resection of the adenoma and, therefore, possible cure. Important predictors of possible surgical cure are location, invasiveness of the tumor, and the preoperative GH levels.

For all other patients, long-acting somatostatin analog treatment should be used. Somatostatin analog is frequently considered as first-line therapy in acromegaly. Biochemical control can be achieved in approximately 50% of patients. When no biochemical control can be achieved with long-acting somatostatin analog treatment, switching to or adding GH receptor antagonist (pegvisomant) is the next step, which can achieve a normal IGF-I level in more than 90% of patients.

Finally, the place for radiotherapy is small and only indicated for those few patients in whom previous interventions did not result in control of tumor size and biochemical activity of the disease. Radiotherapy has significant side effects, such as a progressive decrease in quality of life and increase in hypopituitarism.

For treatment of arthropathy, surgery and treatment with somatostatin analogs was associated with improved symptoms and signs of arthropathy. Treatment effect on cartilage thickness was observed by ultrasonography. Cartilage thickness decreased but did not normalize. Biermasz and colleagues[1] reported that a high prevalence of self-reported joint complaints persisted despite successful long-term treatment of acromegaly.

SUMMARY

Articular involvement in acromegaly is one of the most frequent clinical complications and may be present as the earliest symptom in a significant proportion of patients. The involvement of other organs may be of clinical importance and contribute to increased morbidity and mortality of patients suffered from acromegaly. Early diagnosis and proper treatment of the diseases can prevent the development of irreversible complications of the disease and improve the quality of life in patients suffering from the disease.

REFERENCES

1. Biermasz NR, Pereira AM, Smit JW, et al. Morbidity after long-term remission for acromegaly: persisting joint-related complaints cause reduced quality of life. J Clin Endocrinol Metab 2005;90:2731–9.
2. Wass JA. Acromegaly: a handbook of history, current therapy and future prospect. Bio Scientific Ltd; 2009. p. 43–9.
3. Harris AG. Acromegaly and its management. Philadelphia: Lippincott-Raven; 1996. p. 24–35.
4. Marie P. Sur deux cas d'acromégalie. Rev Med. 1886;6:297–9.
5. Chipman JJ, Attanasio AF, Birkett MA, et al. The safety profile of GH replacement therapy in adults. Clin Endocrinol 1997;46:473–81.
6. Wassenaar MJ, Biermasz NR, van Diunen N, et al. High prevalnece of artropathy, according to the definitions of radiological and clinical osteoarthritis, in patients with long-term cure of acromegaly: a case-control study. Eur J Endocrinol 2009;160:357–65.
7. Podgorski M, Robinson B, Weissberger A, et al. Articular manifestations of acromegaly. Aust N Z J Med 1988;18:28–35.
8. Biermasz NR, van Thiel SW, Pereira AM, et al. Decreased quality of life in patients with acromegaly despite long-term cure of growth hormone excess. J Clin Endocrinol Metab 2004;89:5369–76.
9. Mestron A, Webb SM, Astorga R, et al. Epidemiology, clinical characteristics, outcome, morbidity and mortality in acromegaly based on the Spanish Acromegaly Registry. Eur J Endocrinol 2004;151:439–46.
10. Miller A, Doll H, David J, et al. Impact of musculosceletal disease on quality of life in long-standing acromegaly. Eur J Endocrinol 2008;158:587–93.
11. Kameyama S, Tanaka R, Hasegawa A, et al. Subclinical carpal tunnel syndrome in acromegaly. Neurol Med Chir 1993;33:547–51.
12. Iwasaki N, Masuko T, Ishikawa J, et al. Surgical efficacy of carpal tunnel release for carpal tunnel syndrome in acromegaly: report of four patients. J Hand Surg 2005;6:605–6.
13. Giustina A, Mazziotti G, Canalis A. Growth hormone, insulin-like growth factors and the skeleton. Endocr Rev 2008;29:535–59.

14. Shane E. Osteoporosis associated with illness and medications. In: Marcus R, Feldman D, Relsey J, editors. Osteoporosis. San Diego (CA): Academic Press; 1996. p. 925–46.
15. Bonadonna S, Mazziotti G, Nuzzo M, et al. Increased prevalence of radiological spinal deformities in active acromegaly: a cross- sectional study in postmeno-pausal women. J Bone Miner Res 2005;20:1837–44.
16. Vestergaard P, Mosekilde L. Fracture risk is devreased in acromegaly: a potential beneficial effect of growth hormone. Osteoporos Int 2004;15:155–9.

Hypothalamic-Pituitary-Adrenal Axis in Rheumatoid Arthritis

Richard Imrich, MD, PhD[a,b,*], Jozef Rovenský, MD, DSc, FRCP[c]

KEYWORDS

- Rheumatoid arthritis • Hypothalamic-pituitary-adrenal axis
- Cortisol • Dehydroepiandrosterone
- Adrenocorticotropic hormone
- Corticotropin-releasing hormone • Inflammation • Interleukin-6

The hypothalamic-pituitary-adrenal (HPA) system is a powerful neuroendocrine control mechanism involved in many core body functions including metabolic and energy homeostasis. The HPA axis has been considered an important immune modulator primarily in view of potent anti-inflammatory effects of cortisol in high physiologic and pharmacologic doses. The significance of variations in cortisol concentrations at the lower (unstimulated) normal range for immune regulation is less understood. Conversely, in a controlled environment, administration of systemic mediators of inflammation was found to trigger acute HPA response.[1] Whether the chronic elevation of inflammatory cytokine in patients with inflammatory diseases constitutes an actual HPA stimulus remains a matter of debate. Based on data suggestive of a bi-direction crosstalk between the HPA axis and the immune system, the concept of the neuroendocrine immune (NEI)-negative feedback loop emerged and became a paradigm for studies in autoimmune diseases including rheumatoid arthritis (RA).

This work was supported by grants VEGA 2/0187/09, RASGENAS N00024, NFM/EEA grant SK0095 and CENDO SAV.
The authors have nothing to disclose.
a Center for Molecular Medicine, Slovak Academy of Sciences, Vlarska 3-7, 831 01 Bratislava, Slovak Republic
b Institute of Experimental Endocrinology, Slovak Academy of Sciences, Vlarska 3, 833 06 Bratislava, Slovak Republic
c National Institute of Rheumatic Diseases, Nábrezie Ivana Krasku 4, 92112 Piešťany, Slovakia
* Corresponding author. Center for Molecular Medicine, Slovak Academy of Sciences, Vlarska 3-7, 831 01 Bratislava, Slovak Republic.
E-mail address: richard.imrich@savba.sk

DOES HPA DYSFUNCTION PREDISPOSE TO RA?

Adrenal glucocorticoids, secreted in response to pituitary adrenocorticotropic hormone (ACTH) stimulation, are considered among the key factors involved in regulation of immune responses. Thus dysfunction of the HPA axis has been suspected to be involved in the onset or perpetuation of chronic inflammation in RA. It has been suggested that inherited or acquired down-regulation of the HPA axis essentially would create a predisposing environment for autoimmunity development.[2]

Specific gene variants have been associated with several changes in HPA axis reactivity resulting in suboptimal cortisol levels during challenges.[3] In general, genes involved in HPA function were only rarely studied in association with RA. Corticotrophin-releasing hormone (CRH) promoter polymorphisms were among the first neuroendocrine genes thought to be associated with RA.[4,5] These early studies were performed using the candidate gene approach, and small cohorts had very low statistical power. The association of the CRH promoter polymorphism was not confirmed in subsequent large-scale genome-wide association studies in RA. Similarly, a suspected glucocorticoid receptor polymorphism failed to be confirmed in RA.[6] In addition to genetic predisposition, some early life events appear to program HPA function in adulthood. Thus the process could contribute to development of various diseases including RA as seen in animal models of arthritis.[7,8] Yet, specific data are lacking addressing HPA programming and RA predisposition.

In the context of chronic inflammation, up-regulated HPA function with higher production of cortisol would be anticipated in RA and other inflammatory diseases. Inappropriately low cortisol unable to dampen ongoing inflammation in RA has been conceptualized as a relative adrenal hypofunction.[9,10] Inflammatory cytokines per se were found to have specific effect on adrenal steroids synthesis.[11] Therefore, some of the observed subtle HPA variations could be attributed to ongoing inflammation.

CLINICAL EVIDENCE FOR HPA DYSFUNCTION IN RA

In general, clinical studies in RA demonstrate normal HPA function, which has been considered inappropriately normal for the given level of inflammation.[10] Although subtle differences in endocrine parameters were detected in the clinical studies in RA, their significance for immune system modulation remains unclear.

Interpretations of the inappropriately normal HPA function in RA range from an innate deficiency in the NEI loop effector component, which would be independent of ongoing inflammation, to a direct modulation of endocrine function by inflammatory cytokines.[2,9,11] In addition to HPA axis control mechanisms, synthetic glucocorticoids are used extensively in patients with RA. Recent data suggest efficacy of these drugs in alleviating symptoms of inflammation, and in retarding erosive damage.[12] It becomes clear that the net effect of low-dose glucocorticoids in the treatment of RA favors the beneficial aspects of these drugs over the negative aspects. These clinical findings further reinforce importance of physiologic regulation of the HPA axis in controlling disease activity and progression.

During the past 20 years, a great effort has been made in searching for evidence of improper HPA axis function in RA as demonstrated in animal models of arthritis.[13] In early case-controlled human studies, there were no conclusive differences in urinary corticosteroid metabolites or in corticosteroid secretion in response to ACTH stimulation between RA patients and healthy controls. Neither did circadian secretion of cortisol and ACTH show any differences.[14] Elevated cortisol levels were reported in premenopausal female patients with RA previously not treated with glucocorticoids.[15] On the other hand, another study showed normal serum and normal 24-hour cortisol and elevated ACTH concentrations indicating defective adrenal gland function in untreated RA patients.[16] In a group of 15 patients with clinical symptoms of less than 1 year duration, elevated C-reactive protein and erythrocyte sedimentation rate, and normal cortisol, ACTH, dehydroepiandrosterone (DHEA), and dehydroepiandrosterone sulfate (DHEAS) was observed compared with age- and sex-matched controls.[17] The authors interpreted their findings that in RA patients, the HPA axis is functionally defective already in early stages of the disease, as evidenced by the inappropriately low cortisol levels compared with the ongoing inflammation. In RA patients without prior prednisolone treatment, serum levels of DHEA and cortisol were similar to controls, and serum levels of DHEAS were significantly lower as compared with controls.[18]

The evaluation of HPA axis response to various stimuli yielded controversial results. Chikanza and colleagues[19] showed lower diurnal cortisol levels in RA patients and lower cortisol response to surgical stress as compared with control patients with osteomyelitis and osteoarthritis. Normal results of the CRH stimulation test in these patients indicated normal pituitary and adrenal function. Based on these results, the authors suggested impaired hypothalamic function. The authors also proposed that impaired HPA axis together with observed elevated prolactin levels before and after surgery in RA patients might lead to proinflammatory hormonal status with possible involvement in RA pathogenesis.[19,20] A similar study, however, did not detect differences in ACTH, cortisol, and prolactin levels before and after surgery in RA and osteoarthritis patients.[21]

The insulin-induced hypoglycemia resulted in a minor tendency to lower interval-specific cortisol response in RA patients not treated with glucocorticoids.[22] In a study by Eijsbouts and colleagues,[21] basal plasma and salivary and urinary cortisol levels were not different between patients with RA and healthy controls. During the insulin-induced hypoglycemia, adrenocorticotropic hormone ACTH levels were similar, but cortisol levels were consistently lower in RA patients than in healthy controls.[21] In the authors' controlled investigation of glucocorticoid-naïve premenopausal RA females using the insulin-induced hypoglycemia, basal levels and hypoglycemia-stimulated responses of several adrenal steroids were studied.[23] When compared with age- and body mass index (BMI)-matched healthy females, RA patients had lower basal DHEAS levels and, unexpectedly, a tendency to higher stimulated cortisol response. ACTH response to the hypoglycemia was comparable between RA patients and controls.[23] An evaluation of basal levels of ACTH and cortisol, and subsequent response to CRH stimulation in newly diagnosed RA patients did not detect significant differences compared with healthy controls.[24] Decreased response of DHEA and DHEAS to low-dose ACTH and ovine CRH stimulation in untreated RA females in the follicular phase of the cycle supports the concept that adrenal rather than pituitary function is impaired.[25] Using a bicycle ergometer task, a cold pressor task, and a computerized Stroop color-word interference test as stimuli, RA patients tended to have a less-pronounced ACTH response and had a significantly smaller cortisol response than healthy controls in reaction to the stressors.[26]

CORTISOL KINETICS AND BIOAVAILABILITY IN RA

Evaluation of HPA axis perturbations in RA has been mainly based on an assessment of hormone concentrations in the plasma. An actual concentration of a hormone in plasma depends not only on its secretion but also on the concurrent elimination. As an example, cortisol is metabolized irreversibly by 5-alpha- and 5-beta-reductases to 5-alpha-tetrahydrocortisol and 5-beta-tetrahydrocortisol or converted to biologically inactive cortisone by 11-beta-hydroxysteroid dehydrogenases type 2. Cortisone can be reactivated by 11-beta-hydroxysteroid dehydrogenases type 1 to cortisol or reduced to tetrahydrocortisone by 5-beta-reductase. The authors' group and other groups have studied this aspect of cortisol kinetics in RA. An appropriate approach to study the rate of cortisol distribution and elimination is repeatedly to measure its level in plasma after administration of cortisol in subjects pretreated with dexamethasone to block endogenous cortisol secretion. However, both the authors' study and one by Straub and colleagues failed to detect any differences in cortisol kinetics in RA.[27,28]

The biologically active fraction of cortisol in plasma is the free hormone, which is not bound to plasma proteins. The main binding proteins are cortisol-binding globulin and albumin. The biologically active free fraction of cortisol can be significantly altered by dramatic changes in corticosteroid-binding globulin and albumin, proteins that bind 90% of cortisol in circulation. Severe hypoproteinemia is not typically found in RA patients. However, measurement of free cortisol fraction in serum or salivary cortisol is particularly relevant for adrenal function assessment in subjects on low-dose prednisone, oral contraceptives, or other drugs that interfere with circulating transport proteins of cortisol. Inflammatory cytokines in RA also may affect elastase-induced cleavage of cortisol from its transport proteins, thus affecting cortisol availability in local tissues.[29] Recently, the authors compared cortisol responses to the low-dose (1 μg) ACTH test in a group of RA females on low-dose prednisone/methylprednisolone (<8 mg/d), glucocorticoid-naïve RA females, and in age- and BMI-matched healthy females. In addition to measuring total plasma cortisol, the authors also measured free cortisol response to ACTH. Total plasma cortisol responses to ACTH were lower in both glucocorticoid-naïve and glucocorticoid untreated RA patients compared with matched controls. Interestingly, free cortisol response to ACTH, however, did not differ between glucocorticoid-naïve RA subjects and controls, while the free cortisol response to ACTH was significantly lower in the prednisone-treated RA patients compared with healthy controls (Imrich, unpublished observations, 2010). This study demonstrates that significance of total cortisol measurements can be in some cases misleading in terms of real cortisol bioavailability.

ADRENAL ANDROGENS IN RA

Most physiologic attention had previously been given to the tropic (stimulation) aspects in the HPA negative feedback signaling system.[30] Little attention has been given to considerations of trophic (cell mass/competence) influences, which may apply, particularly at the adrenal gland level.[31] Specifically, adrenal glands of premenopausal-onset RA patients or susceptibles may have relatively deficient mass capacity of their endocrine function, particularly of the zona reticularis production of adrenal androgens.[32] Mechanisms regulating the dissociation of glucocorticoids and adrenal androgens remain unclear. These may involve functional and anatomic changes in the zona reticularis of the adrenals.

Evaluation of androgen concentrations in RA patients showed decreased DHEAS in premenopausal women and decreased testosterone levels in men.[9] A study of 50 human leukocyte antigen (HLA) identical postmenopausal RA discordant sibling pairs revealed significantly lower levels of DHEAS in the RA siblings, and their DHEAS levels correlated with disease severity and duration.[33] A prospective study showed decreased DHEAS levels in 35 women before disease development.[9] A similar study in Finland reported no significant differences between 116 patients and 329 controls.[34]

The reasons for these discrepant results include differences in methodology or in genetic factors. The observed decreased plasma concentrations of adrenal androgens may be due to lower pooling, lower sensitivity to ACTH, or an enzymatic defect of the adrenals. Patients previously not treated with glucocorticoids have changed steroidogenesis of DHEA and DHEAS.[25]

Combined lower DHEAS and lower baseline cortisol levels could indicate adrenocortical hypocompetence, yet not be clinically apparent. In their previous study, the authors identified about 40% of premenopausal RA females with combined relatively lower basal cortisol and lower DHEAS.[35,36] This result might suggest decreased basal adrenal function in a subset of RA patients that involves both the glucocorticoid-producing zona fasciculata and the androgen-producing zona reticularis.

SUMMARY

The controlled data accumulated so far support only subtle alterations in HPA axis function in RA, mainly at the adrenal level, and particularly in a subset of premenopausal-onset women. Such interpretation is supported by consistent findings of lower levels of adrenal androgens, particularly DHEAS, in premenopausal-onset RA patients. Consequences of the subtle HPA alterations in RA for the disease development remain unclear. From a broader perspective, the unresponsiveness of the HPA axis to chronic inflammation in RA simply can be seen as an ongoing adaptation to the disease state with higher priority to proper regulation of core body functions over the immune homeostasis.

REFERENCES

1. Mastorakos G, Weber JS, Magiakou MA, et al. Hypothalamic-pituitary-adrenal axis activation and stimulation of systemic vasopressin secretion by recombinant interleukin-6 in humans: potential implications for the syndrome of inappropriate vasopressin secretion. J Clin Endocrinol Metab 1994;79:934.
2. Masi AT, Aldag JC. Integrated neuroendocrine immune risk factors in relation to rheumatoid arthritis: should rheumatologists now adopt a model of a multiyear, presymptomatic phase? Scand J Rheumatol 2005;34:342.
3. Derijk RH. Single nucleotide polymorphisms related to HPA axis reactivity. Neuro-immunomodulation 2009;16:340.
4. Baerwald CG, Mok CC, Tickly M, et al. Corticotropin releasing hormone (CRH) promoter polymorphisms in various ethnic groups of patients with rheumatoid arthritis. Z Rheumatol 2000;59:29.
5. Fife M, Steer S, Fisher S, et al. Association of familial and sporadic rheumatoid arthritis with a single corticotropin-releasing hormone genomic region (8q12.3) haplotype. Arthritis Rheum 2002;46:75.
6. Donn R, Payne D, Ray D. Glucocorticoid receptor gene polymorphisms and susceptibility to rheumatoid arthritis. Clin Endocrinol (Oxf) 2007;67:342.
7. Levitt NS, Lambert EV, Woods D, et al. Impaired glucose tolerance and elevated blood pressure in low birth weight, nonobese, young South African adults: early programming of cortisol axis. J Clin Endocrinol Metab 2000;85:4611.
8. Lightman SL, Windle RJ, Ma XM, et al. Hypothalamic-pituitary-adrenal function. Arch Physiol Biochem 2002;110:90.
9. Masi AT. Sex hormones and rheumatoid arthritis: cause or effect relationships in a complex pathophysiology? Clin Exp Rheumatol 1995;13:227.
10. Straub RH, Paimela L, Peltomaa R, et al. Inadequately low serum levels of steroid hormones in relation to interleukin-6 and tumor necrosis factor in untreated

patients with early rheumatoid arthritis and reactive arthritis. Arthritis Rheum 2002;46:654.

11. Herrmann M, Scholmerich J, Straub RH. Influence of cytokines and growth factors on distinct steroidogenic enzymes in vitro: a short tabular data collection. Ann N Y Acad Sci 2002;966:166.

12. Hoes JN, Jacobs JWG, Buttgereit F, et al. Current view of glucocorticoid cotherapy in rheumatoid arthritis. Nat Rev Rheumatol 2010, in press.

13. Sternberg EM, Hill JM, Chrousos GP, et al. Inflammatory mediator-induced hypothalamic-pituitary-adrenal axis activation is defective in streptococcal cell wall arthritis-susceptible Lewis rats. Proc Natl Acad Sci U S A 1989;86:2374.

14. Harkness JA, Richter MB, Panayi GS, et al. Circadian variation in disease activity in rheumatoid arthritis. Br Med J (Clin Res Ed) 1982;284:551.

15. Mirone L, Altomonte L, D'Agostino P, et al. A study of serum androgen and cortisol levels in female patients with rheumatoid arthritis. Correlation with disease activity. Clin Rheumatol 1996;15:15.

16. Gudbjornsson B, Skogseid B, Oberg K, et al. Intact adrenocorticotropic hormone secretion but impaired cortisol response in patients with active rheumatoid arthritis. Effect of glucocorticoids. J Rheumatol 1996;23:596.

17. Kanik KS, Chrousos GP, Schumacher HR, et al. Adrenocorticotropin, glucocorticoid, and androgen secretion in patients with new onset synovitis/rheumatoid arthritis: relations with indices of inflammation. J Clin Endocrinol Metab 2000;85:1461.

18. Vogl D, Falk W, Dorner M, et al. Serum levels of pregnenolone and 17-hydroxy-pregnenolone in patients with rheumatoid arthritis and systemic lupus erythematosus: relation to other adrenal hormones. J Rheumatol 2003;30:269.

19. Chikanza IC, Petrou P, Kingsley G, et al. Defective hypothalamic response to immune and inflammatory stimuli in patients with rheumatoid arthritis. Arthritis Rheum 1992;35:1281.

20. Chikanza IC, Petrou P, Chrousos G, et al. Excessive and dysregulated secretion of prolactin in rheumatoid arthritis: immunopathogenetic and therapeutic implications. Br J Rheumatol 1993;32:445.

21. Eijsbouts A, van den Hoogen F, Laan R, et al. Similar response of adrenocorticotropic hormone, cortisol and prolactin to surgery in rheumatoid arthritis and osteoarthritis. Br J Rheumatol 1998;37:1138.

22. Gutierrez MA, Garcia ME, Rodriguez JA, et al. Hypothalamic-pituitary-adrenal axis function in patients with active rheumatoid arthritis: a controlled study using insulin hypoglycemia stress test and prolactin stimulation. J Rheumatol 1999;26:277.

23. Imrich R, Rovensky J, Malis F, et al. Low levels of dehydroepiandrosterone sulphate in plasma, and reduced sympathoadrenal response to hypoglycaemia in premenopausal women with rheumatoid arthritis. Ann Rheum Dis 2005;64:202.

24. Templ E, Koeller M, Riedl M, et al. Anterior pituitary function in patients with newly diagnosed rheumatoid arthritis. Br J Rheumatol 1996;35:350.

25. Cutolo M, Foppiani L, Prete C, et al. Hypothalamic-pituitary-adrenocortical axis function in premenopausal women with rheumatoid arthritis not treated with glucocorticoids. J Rheumatol 1999;26:282.

26. Dekkers JC, Geenen R, Godaert GL, et al. Experimentally challenged reactivity of the hypothalamic pituitary adrenal axis in patients with recently diagnosed rheumatoid arthritis. J Rheumatol 2001;28:1496.

27. Straub RH, Weidler C, Demmel B, et al. Renal clearance and daily excretion of cortisol and adrenal androgens in patients with rheumatoid arthritis and systemic lupus erythematosus. Ann Rheum Dis 2004;63:961.

28. Rovensky J, Imrich R, Koska J, et al. Cortisol elimination from plasma in premenopausal women with rheumatoid arthritis. Ann Rheum Dis 2003;62:674.

29. Pemberton PA, Stein PE, Pepys MB, et al. Hormone binding globulins undergo serpin conformational change in inflammation. Nature 1988;336:257.

30. Watts AG. Glucocorticoid regulation of peptide genes in neuroendocrine CRH neurons: a complexity beyond negative feedback. Front Neuroendocrinol 2005; 26:109.

31. Masi AT, Da Silva JA, Cutolo M. Perturbations of hypothalamic-pituitary-gonadal (HPG) axis and adrenal androgen (AA) functions in rheumatoid arthritis. Baillieres Clin Rheumatol 1996;10:295.

32. Imrich R, Vlcek M, Aldag JC, et al. An endocrinologist's view on relative adrenocortical insufficiency in rheumatoid arthritis. Ann N Y Acad Sci 2010;1193:134.

33. Deighton CM, Watson MJ, Walker DJ. Sex hormones in postmenopausal HLA-identical rheumatoid arthritis discordant sibling pairs. J Rheumatol 1992;19:1663.

34. Heikkila R, Aho K, Heliovaara M, et al. Serum androgen–anabolic hormones and the risk of rheumatoid arthritis. Ann Rheum Dis 1998;57:281.

35. Cebecauer L, Radikova Z, Rovensky J, et al. Increased prevalence and coincidence of antinuclear and antithyroid antibodies in the population exposed to high levels of polychlorinated pollutants cocktail. Endocr Regul 2009;43:75.

36. Imrich R, Vigas M, Rovensky J, et al. Adrenal plasma steroid relations in glucocorticoid-naive premenopausal rheumatoid arthritis patients during insulin-induced hypoglycemia test compared to matched normal control females. Endocr Regul 2009;43:65.

Rheumatologic Manifestations of Pregnancy

Lisa R. Sammaritano, MD

KEYWORDS

- Pregnancy • Rheumatologic manifestations
- Musculoskeletal symptoms • Tenosynovitis
- Carpal tunnel syndrome • Preeclampsia

Normal pregnancy induces profound multisystemic changes similar in magnitude to those seen in many well-defined endocrine disorders. However, unlike other endocrine conditions, pregnancy may affect up to half of the normal population. Alterations in the reproductive hormones persist through pregnancy and the initial postpartum period and affect the maternal anatomy, physiology, and metabolism. Familiarity with hormone-induced changes is critical to differentiate between normal and abnormal pregnancy manifestations as well as to differentiate between pregnancy-related symptoms and possible rheumatic disease. Rheumatic diseases disproportionately affect women, often presenting during the childbearing years. Changes of normal and abnormal pregnancy may mimic various symptoms of rheumatologic diseases, including musculoskeletal, dermatologic, hematologic, renal, and neurologic manifestations. The converse may also be true: the initial onset of rheumatologic disorders during pregnancy may present great difficulty in diagnosis because symptoms may be erroneously attributed to normal or complicated pregnancy, delaying appropriate diagnosis and therapy and ultimately affecting prognosis.

MUSCULOSKELETAL MANIFESTATIONS OF PREGNANCY

Musculoskeletal complaints are frequent in pregnancy. Normal changes of ligamentous laxity, soft tissue edema, weight gain, and alteration in the center of gravity contribute to the musculoskeletal symptoms associated with pregnancy. Ligamentous laxity is an important physiologic change of pregnancy, allowing remodeling of the pelvic architecture and widening of the symphysis pubis to permit transvaginal passage of the fetus. Soft tissue edema is noted in up to 80% of women, most commonly during the last 8 weeks of pregnancy, and can contribute to tenosynovial

The author has nothing to disclose.

Rheumatology Division, Department of Medicine, Hospital for Special Surgery, Weill Cornell Medical College, 535 East 70th Street, New York, NY 10021, USA

E-mail address: Sammaritan@hss.edu

Rheum Dis Clin N Am 36 (2010) 729–740

doi:10.1016/j.rdc.2010.09.006

rheumatic.theclinics.com

or nerve entrapment.[1] Weight gain places additional stress on joints: a 20% increase in weight during pregnancy can increase the force on a joint by as much as 100%.[2] The position of the gravid uterus shifts the center of gravity, causing hyperlordosis, which contributes to the mechanical strain on the back and sacroiliac joints.

It has been suggested that pelvic and low-back pain of pregnancy is related to pregnancy-related hormones in addition to the altered biomechanical forces. Although ligamentous laxity was initially attributed to the production of the pregnancy hormone relaxin,[3] more recent evidence does not support a strict correlation with the relaxin level,[4] that is, relaxin level increases until peaking at 12 weeks, followed by a decline with stabilization at week 17 at 50% of the peak level.[3] Estrogen may be more important for laxity. A small study evaluating 40 knees in 20 pregnant patients showed that high serum estradiol levels during the third trimester correlated with increased anterior tibial translation, measured serially during pregnancy and postpartum. The degree of translation decreased as the serum estradiol returned to nonpregnant levels during the postpartum period.[5]

Low-Back and Pelvic Pain

Up to 72% of pregnant women complain of back pain during the course of pregnancy.[6] Risk of low-back pain increases with an advancing maternal age, a history of previous pregnancy-related low-back pain, multiparity, a higher body mass index, and a history of hypermobility.[7] Exercise before and during pregnancy may be protective.[7,8] Contributing factors include mechanical strain, pelvic ligamentous laxity, sacroiliac pain, vascular compression, and spondylolisthesis.[9] True lumbar radiculopathy as a cause of pregnancy-associated low-back pain is atypical, occurring in about 1% of pregnant women.[10] Cauda equina syndrome resulting from lumbar disk herniation is rarer but reported and is estimated to occur in 1 in 10,000 pregnant women.[11] Classic symptoms include bilateral radicular leg pain with bladder or bowel dysfunction and saddle anesthesia; if neurologic symptoms progress, surgery may be indicated during pregnancy.

Pelvic girdle pain of pregnancy is common and may affect the anterior or posterior pelvis. Pain in the pubic symphysis usually occurs because of increased motion as a result of ligamentous laxity. The syndrome of osteitis pubis is characterized by a gradual onset of pubic symphysis pain followed by rapid progression over several days to severe pain radiating down the inner thighs; although painful, recovery generally occurs within several days to weeks. The syndrome is also characterized by bony resorption about the symphysis followed by spontaneous reossification and may occur during pregnancy or in the postpartum period. Spontaneous rupture of the pubic symphysis, with complete tear of the ligaments, is rare and occurs most commonly during parturition. This rupture is believed to be caused by the forceful descent of the fetal head against the pelvic ring.[12] Treatment is usually conservative with bed rest, pelvic support, and pain control, although surgical fixation is occasionally required.[13] True pelvic dislocation because of the rupture of the symphysis pubis as well as the sacroiliac joint ligaments is extremely rare and is best managed with a surgical approach.[14]

Osteitis condensans ilii is a radiologic diagnosis identified on radiograph in the postpartum period during workup for back or pelvic pain, which can be confused with inflammatory sacroiliitis. It is a benign, but sometimes painful condition, characterized by bilateral and symmetric sclerosis (triangular) on the iliac side of the sacroiliac joints; unlike sacroiliitis associated with ankylosing spondylitis and other inflammatory conditions, articular margins are intact and the joint space is preserved. The condition is most common in multiparous women and may result from mechanical stress across the sacroiliac joints in association with other pregnancy changes. Most affected women note the onset of pain during pregnancy or the postpartum period. Therapy is conservative with physical therapy and analgesics; radiographic results often return to normal over time.[15,16]

Hip Pain

True hip pain, as distinct from hip area pain radiating from the back or pelvis, is an uncommon but concerning symptom during pregnancy. The differential diagnosis includes transient osteoporosis and avascular necrosis of the hip. Transient osteoporosis of the hip usually presents during the third trimester. This osteoporosis is a self-limiting demineralization of the femoral head and neck, which spontaneously resolves over 6 months. The typical presentation is the onset of acute hip pain worsened by weight bearing and relieved with rest.[17] Prognosis is good if recognized; if not diagnosed, continued weight bearing may lead to fracture.[18] Although usually unilateral, bilateral involvement leading to bilateral femoral neck and acetabular fractures has been reported.[19] Treatment with antiresorptive bone agents such as calcitonin and bisphosphonates may shorten symptom duration in pregnant and postpartum patients,[20,21] although use of bisphosphonates during pregnancy is controversial and is generally discouraged.

Avascular necrosis of the hip has been reported in pregnant patients who do not have other predisposing factors.[22] The clinical presentation may be similar to that of transient osteoporosis of the hip, with pain exacerbated by weight bearing, often during the third trimester. Prognosis is variable, and postpartum core decompression or hip replacement may be necessary.[17] Magnetic resonance imaging can effectively distinguish between transient osteoporosis and avascular necrosis and is considered safe in pregnancy.[23]

Tenosynovitis

de Quervain tenosynovitis is the inflammation of the abductor pollicis longus and extensor pollicis brevis tendons in the first dorsal compartment of the wrist. Although often related to repetitive movement, this condition is also common in pregnant and lactating women. Patients develop pain with thumb movement, which radiates to the radial aspect of the wrist. Finkelstein test is diagnostic, with pain provoked by ulnar flexion of the closed fist with the thumb inside. Occurrence during pregnancy and lactation is attributed to fluid retention associated with hormonal changes. During the postpartum period, it may also be because of child care. Pregnancy- and postpartum-related disease is self-limited and usually resolves with cessation of pregnancy or lactation.[24] Treatment during pregnancy or lactation includes splinting and/or corticosteroid injection. In one small study, corticosteroid injection was more effective than splinting and so may be the preferred temporizing therapy.[25]

Arthralgia and Arthritis

In addition to the common musculoskeletal manifestations of pregnancy, otherwise healthy women may also complain of small joint pain during pregnancy, raising the question of inflammatory disease, such as systemic lupus erythematosus (SLE) or rheumatoid arthritis. Choi and colleagues[26] recently evaluated the incidence of arthritis and arthralgia in a series of 155 healthy pregnant women followed up at Seoul National University Hospital between January and May 2004. Patients with other musculoskeletal diagnoses were excluded, including those with low-back pain, pelvic girdle pain, symphysis pubis pain, hip pain, carpal tunnel syndrome, rheumatic disease, trauma, or infection. Patients were evaluated by rheumatologists serially throughout pregnancy and for 6 weeks postpartum. The frequency of arthralgia was

16.7% and that of arthritis was 9.6%. Arthralgia and arthritis usually developed in the third trimester, and the proximal interphalangeal joints were most commonly involved. In most cases, symptoms improved spontaneously. Although one patient later developed spondyloarthropathy, no patient developed rheumatoid arthritis or SLE during the follow-up period. Symptoms were attributed to the characteristic changes in edema, joint laxity, hormone levels, and cytokines seen in pregnancy.[26]

Onset of new rheumatoid arthritis during pregnancy is unusual, and studies suggest that pregnancy is protective against new-onset rheumatoid disease. However, an increased risk of disease onset is noted in the postpartum period.[27] As a result, new onset of polyarthralgia or polyarthritis in the postpartum period should raise concerns about a new diagnosis of rheumatoid arthritis.

CUTANEOUS MANIFESTATIONS OF PREGNANCY

Physiologic skin changes induced by pregnancy are primarily of cosmetic concern. However, these changes may mimic those suggesting flare of existing rheumatic disease or prompt concern about a new rheumatic disease diagnosis. Changes are seen in pigmentation, hair growth, nails, glandular function, connective tissues of the skin, and vascular structures.

Pigment Changes

Hyperpigmentation occurs in up to 90% of pregnant women. Melasma (chloasma or mask of pregnancy) is a diffuse macular facial hyperpigmentation found in up to 70% of pregnant women.[28] A malar distribution, mimicking a lupus rash, is most common, followed by a more generalized facial distribution (centrofacial pattern). Like rash associated with lupus, symptoms are often exacerbated by exposure to visible and ultraviolet light. Melasma is more common in those with darker baseline skin tone.[29] Although the change usually resolves postpartum, it may persist in darker-skinned individuals and often recurs in subsequent pregnancies or with the use of oral contraceptives. Despite the malar distribution and sun sensitivity, true inflammatory changes, such as those associated with lupus rash, are not seen.

Vascular Changes

Blood flow to the skin increases significantly by the end of the second month of pregnancy because of elevated estrogen levels and increased blood volume. Spider angiomas and telangiectasias develop in up to two-thirds of White women, usually resolving in the postpartum period.[30] Nonpitting edema is frequent and may occur early owing to hormonal factors. These changes may suggest skin abnormalities associated with the systemic sclerosis spectrum of disease. Palmar erythema is seen in 30% to 70% of women, and when prominent, it may mimic cutaneous vasculitis seen in SLE or other connective tissue diseases.

Other Changes

A common pregnancy-induced dermatologic change suggestive of connective tissue disease is postpartum hair loss (telogen effluvium), which can be noticeable and distressing even when expected. Although usually limited to a period of several months, the hair loss may take up to 15 months to resolve, prompting concern about an underlying process. Before delivery, some women note a less-typical frontoparietal hair recession and diffuse hair thinning in the later months of pregnancy.[31] Nail changes may occur, including onycholysis, grooving, and subungual hyperkeratosis. These changes may suggest psoriatic arthritis, especially in the setting of the common pregnancy complaint of low-back pain. Pruritis and urticaria also occur in pregnancy, which are nonspecific symptoms that may also present in connective tissue and other systemic diseases.

Pregnancy-Associated Rashes

Uncommon dermatoses specific to pregnancy may be confused with new-onset auto-immune rashes. Uncommon dermatoses include autoimmune progesterone dermatitis, pruritic urticarial papules and plaques of pregnancy, impetigo herpetiformis (a form of pustular psoriasis), and herpes gestationis (which shares many features with bullous pemphigoid but is limited to pregnant women). It is especially important to appropriately identify impetigo herpetiformis and herpes gestationis because they may be associated with the risk of maternal or fetal adverse effects.[31]

Erythema Nodosum

Erythema nodosum is an acute nodular erythematous eruption on the extensor aspect of the lower legs; pathologic study shows a septal panniculitis without evidence of vasculitis. Erythema nodosum likely represents a hypersensitivity response to an unknown antigen (or antigens); its presence prompts workup for underlying rheumatic disease or infection. Common causes include streptococcal infection, tuberculosis, drugs (including oral contraceptives), sarcoidosis, Behçet syndrome, and enteropathies.[32] Pregnancy is an uncommon but well-recognized cause of erythema nodosum, accounting for 2% of patients in a recent series of 100 patients.[33] Recurrence of erythema nodosum in subsequent pregnancies and with the use of oral contraceptives has been reported.[34,35]

HEMATOLOGIC MANIFESTATIONS OF PREGNANCY

Blood volume increases by 40% to 50% during pregnancy, resulting from an increase in both plasma volume and red blood cell mass. However, the increase in plasma volume is proportionally greater than that of the red blood cell mass, and so maternal hematocrit falls during normal pregnancy, causing physiologic anemia[36] that may exacerbate or mimic anemia of chronic disease.

Most studies confirm a mild decrease in platelet count within the normal range during gestation, which is attributed to increased destruction and hemodilution.[37] About 8% of pregnant women develop a more significant decrease in platelet count, termed gestational thrombocytopenia, in the third trimester with platelet counts between 70,000 and 150,000/mm^3, which is attributed to an acceleration of the usual increased platelet consumption associated with pregnancy.[38] Counts return to normal within several weeks postpartum. Infants are rarely born with below-normal counts. Although gestational thrombocytopenia is not associated with maternal or perinatal complications, it may be confused with autoimmune thrombocytopenia or preeclampsia.

White blood cell (WBC) count increases slightly during pregnancy because of an increase in circulating neutrophils, and counts markedly increase from 20 to 30,000/mm^3 during labor, making WBC count less useful as an indicator of inflammation. The immune system changes overall during pregnancy to allow maternal tolerance of the fetus, resulting in a decrease in cell-mediated cytotoxic immune responses and an increase in humeral and innate responses. The decrease in cellular immunity leads to an increased susceptibility to intracellular pathogens. Serum complement levels are normal or slightly increased; as a result, these levels are less reliable in diagnosing or ruling out autoimmune disease activity.[36]

Profound changes occur in the coagulation system during pregnancy and in combination with increased venous stasis, compression by the gravid uterus, and bed rest, which significantly increase the risk of thromboembolism during pregnancy and the postpartum period. Overall risk of thromboembolism in pregnancy is 1 per 1500, increased by a factor of 5.[39] Most procoagulant factors increase, including fibrinogen and factors VII, IX, and X, whereas protein S levels decrease. The increase in fibrinogen is associated with an increase in the erythrocyte sedimentation rate (ESR), so that it is no longer useful as an indicator of inflammation.[36]

Hematologic Complications

Although gestational thrombocytopenia is the most common cause of a low platelet count in pregnancy, less common conditions may also cause thrombocytopenia and, unlike gestational thrombocytopenia, can be associated with maternal and perinatal morbidity. These common conditions include immune thrombocytopenic purpura (ITP), severe preeclampsia, HELLP (hemolysis, elevated liver enzymes, and low platelet count occurring in association with preeclampsia) syndrome, and disseminated intravascular coagulation (DIC); rarer causes include antiphospholipid syndrome (APS), SLE, thrombotic thrombocytopenic purpura (TTP), and hemolytic uremic syndrome (HUS).[40] Platelet antibody testing cannot distinguish among gestational thrombocytopenia, ITP, and preeclampsia, although the antibodies associated with gestational thrombocytopenia may not be specific antiplatelet antibodies.[41]

Idiopathic thrombocytopenic purpura, although affecting only 3 in 1000 pregnancies, is of concern because profound neonatal thrombocytopenia may occur in infants; incidence of platelet count less than 50,000/mm^3 ranges from 5% to 38%. Despite the high incidence of low counts, neonatal complications are unusual and the mode of delivery does not seem to affect the outcome.[40] Reported neonatal complications include intraventricular hemorrhage, hemopericardium, gastrointestinal bleeding, and cutaneous bleeding.[41]

TTP and HUS are characterized by microangiopathic hemolytic anemia and severe thrombocytopenia. TTP is characterized by the presence of the hematologic abnormalities in combination with neurologic abnormalities, fever, and renal insufficiency and may be easily confused with, or occur in combination with, SLE or catastrophic APS. Seven percent of TTP cases are reported to occur during pregnancy or the postpartum period.[42] In a series of 45 reported cases of TTP in pregnancy, 40 patients developed the disease antepartum, with 50% occurring before 24 weeks' gestation.[43] In contrast, HUS, which is characterized by more severe renal disease, usually has its onset in the postpartum period but may also be confused with postpartum preeclampsia, lupus nephritis, or vasculitis.

HELLP Syndrome

HELLP syndrome is identified by the triad of hemolysis (microangiopathic hemolytic anemia), elevated liver function tests, and low platelet count. HELLP syndrome is considered to be a variant of severe preeclampsia, but hypertension and proteinuria need not be present.[44] Commonly associated symptoms include right upper quadrant or epigastric pain, nausea and vomiting, and headache. Severe associated complications include multiorgan dysfunction, DIC, liver infarction or hemorrhage, adult respiratory distress syndrome, and acute renal failure. Clinical findings may mimic severe gastrointestinal illness, ITP, SLE, TTP, and HUS. Therapy is determined by the gestational stage and clinical severity of presentation and may include immediate delivery or expectant management with plasma volume expansion, antithrombotic agents, corticosteroid, fresh frozen plasma, and plasmapheresis. Maternal mortality is estimated at 1% and the rates of morbidity are high. It was reported that 30% of cases develop in the postpartum period, most of these within 48 hours of delivery.[45] The onset of HELLP in the second trimester has been associated with underlying APS.[46,47] Early or severe presentation of HELLP, especially with liver infarction, should prompt evaluation for underlying APS or other connective tissue disease.

CARDIOVASCULAR MANIFESTATIONS OF PREGNANCY

Cardiac output increases greatly during pregnancy because of the concomitant increase in plasma volume, starting in early pregnancy, peaking at 30% to 50% above normal levels[48] and providing additional stress for patients with preexisting cardiac compromise. Both components of cardiac output, stroke volume and heart rate, increase. Although the heart size does not change during pregnancy, the heart rotates and moves upward because of the displacement by the raised diaphragm, moving the apex laterally and resulting in an increased cardiac silhouette on the chest radiograph.[36] Despite the increase in cardiac output, maternal blood pressure decreases from baseline until late in pregnancy because of a decrease in systemic vascular resistance. Pregnancy-related exertional dyspnea is common, usually beginning before 20 weeks. Other normal symptoms may include fatigue, occasional orthopnea, syncope, and chest discomfort. Normal findings on examination include peripheral edema, tachycardia, jugular venous distention, altered heart sounds, new systolic and diastolic murmurs, and a new continuous murmur in the second to fourth intercostal space caused by increased blood flow in the breast.[49]

Cardiac Complications

Gestational hypertension develops in previously normotensive women after 20 weeks of pregnancy and resolves within 3 months postpartum. Risk of progression to severe hypertension, preeclampsia, and eclampsia is increased with lower gestational age at the time of diagnosis[50]; overall, 10% to 25% of patients with gestational hypertension progress to overt preeclampsia.[51]

Peripartum cardiomyopathy (PPCM) is a rare syndrome of idiopathic cardiomyopathy occurring in the last month of pregnancy or up to 5 months postpartum. Immediate mortality rate is 9% to 25%, but more than half of the women with PPCM recover, with normal heart size, and function within 6 months of delivery.[52] Complete recovery is more likely in women with a left ventricular ejection fraction of more than 30% at diagnosis. The rest of the women experience either persistent stable left ventricular dysfunction or gradual clinical deterioration.[53] Although cardiomyopathy in young women is rare, it may also be a manifestation of connective tissue disease, such as SLE or inflammatory myositis.

RENAL MANIFESTATIONS OF PREGNANCY

Glomerular filtration rate increases early, by 5 to 7 weeks gestation, and is 50% higher than prepregnancy values by the end of the first trimester. This elevated filtration rate is maintained until the end of pregnancy and returns to normal by 3 months postpartum.[36] Patients with preexisting renal insufficiency may have difficulty tolerating or accommodating to the increased renal filtration, and further deterioration in renal function may occur as a result of hemodynamic stress. In a normal pregnancy, maternal hyperfiltration results in a reduction in maternal creatinine, blood urea nitrogen, and uric acid. No significant increase in proteinuria occurs during normal pregnancy in women without preexisting proteinuria.[54] However, in those women with preexisting proteinuria, the level of urinary protein increases in the second and third trimesters to about twice the baseline values.[55] Although the presence of microscopic hematuria during pregnancy suggests concern for nephritis or other pathologic conditions, up to 16% of pregnant women may have microscopic hematuria due to increased vascular tortuousity in the bladder.[56]

Renal Complications

Preeclampsia is characterized by new-onset hypertension (blood pressure >140/90 mm Hg) with proteinuria (>300 mg per 24 hours) and edema after 20 weeks' gestation. It affects 2% to 7% of healthy nulliparous women; risk is increased in women with preexisting renal disease, multifetal gestation, hypertension, previous preeclampsia, diabetes mellitus, and thrombophilias, including APS. Serum creatinine is rarely increased, but uric acid is commonly elevated. Thrombocytopenia occurs in up to half of the patients with severe preeclampsia.[57]

Preeclampsia may be difficult to differentiate from acute onset of rheumatologic disease, including lupus nephritis, scleroderma renal crisis, and polyarteritis nodosa (PAN). For example, thrombocytopenia, hypertension, proteinuria, and hyperuricemia occur in both lupus nephritis and preeclampsia. ESR and complement levels are often unhelpful because of pregnancy-related changes. Clinical signs that point toward a new diagnosis or exacerbation of connective tissue disease include inflammatory arthritis (as opposed to arthralgia), inflammatory rash (as opposed to vascular erythema), fever, lymphadenopathy, hematuria, leukopenia, red blood cell casts, and positive antinuclear and anti–double-stranded DNA antibodies. Very early or severe preeclampsia should prompt consideration of underlying diagnoses; for example, APS predisposes to early and severe preeclampsia and HELLP syndrome.[46] Rare diseases may be difficult to diagnose when presenting during pregnancy, which may delay appropriate therapy. As an example, PAN is most common in middle-aged men and does not typically present in young women. Of the 7 cases of PAN reported during pregnancy, all patients presented either during late pregnancy or the postpartum period, and all died by postpartum day 42. Diagnosis was made at autopsy for 6 of 7 patients, which revealed that hypertension and renal insufficiency were initially attributed to preeclampsia rather than the new onset of a rare autoimmune disease.[58]

NEUROLOGIC MANIFESTATIONS OF PREGNANCY
Carpal Tunnel Syndrome

Compression of the median nerve may occur during pregnancy because of edema and weight gain, resulting in carpal tunnel syndrome. Prevalence is 2% to 3%, and risk is greatest in primigravidas older than 30 years.[59] Onset is most common during the third trimester, and symptoms usually resolve within 2 weeks of delivery. Onset in the postpartum period is associated with breastfeeding.[60] Conservative treatment with splinting is usually effective[59]; corticosteroid injection may be helpful, and the need for surgical release is uncommon. Overall prognosis is good, although recent long-term follow-up of a series of women with carpal tunnel syndrome during pregnancy showed that half of the women still had some symptoms 3 years after delivery, and 11% still wore night splints; however, only 1 of 45 women underwent surgery at 5 months postpartum. Despite the improvement in symptoms, distal sensory conduction velocity of the median nerve was delayed to some extent in 84% of women at 1 year after delivery.[61]

Other Neuropathies

Other compressive neuropathies may also be associated with pregnancy or labor and delivery, including meralgia paresthetica (lateral femoral cutaneous neuropathy), femoral neuropathy, and lumbosacral plexopathies.

Chorea Gravidarum

Chorea gravidarum is the presentation of chorea during pregnancy. Causes may be variable, including underlying movement disorder such as Huntington disease, rheumatic fever (Sydenham chorea), SLE, APS, or idiopathic condition. Chorea gravidarum most often presents during the second to fifth month of pregnancy but has also presented during the postpartum period. The condition usually resolves within weeks to months of delivery but may reoccur in subsequent pregnancies or with the use of oral contraceptives.[62,63] Chorea has also been associated with APS and SLE, independent of pregnancy.[64]

Eclampsia

Eclampsia is the occurrence of seizures or coma unrelated to other cerebral conditions with signs and symptoms of preeclampsia; incidence is about 1 in 2000 pregnancies. In addition to hypertension, proteinuria, and edema, other clinical symptoms include occipital or frontal headache, blurred vision, photophobia, epigastric or right upper quadrant pain, and altered mental status.[65] The frequency of postpartum eclampsia ranges from 11% to 44%, and occurrence may be as late as 23 days postpartum.[66] Late presentation or presentation without typical signs of preeclampsia, such as hypertension or proteinuria, may lead to consideration of alternative diagnoses, including neuropsychiatric SLE or central nervous system vasculitis.

GASTROINTESTINAL MANIFESTATIONS OF PREGNANCY

Pregnancy is associated with hormone-mediated decreased motility in the esophagus, stomach, and small intestine; a decreased risk of peptic ulcer disease; and an increase in gastroesophageal reflux disease and dyspepsia.[36] Constipation is common (11%–38%), although diarrhea may also occur.[67] Decreased motility and increased reflux may exacerbate or mimic motility disorders of connective tissue diseases, especially systemic sclerosis.

SUMMARY

Pregnancy, whether normal or complicated, induces change in nearly every system of the body. Because most rheumatologic disorders are multisystemic and often affect young women, it may be difficult to differentiate pregnancy-related change from new onset or exacerbation of rheumatic disease. Familiarity with common manifestations of pregnancy is important in evaluating young women of childbearing age, whether or not they have known rheumatologic disease. Presentation of new connective tissue disease during pregnancy is often associated with poorer prognosis, so it is especially important to distinguish between pregnancy-induced change and true autoimmune inflammation requiring prompt and aggressive therapy.

REFERENCES

1. Borg-Stein J, Dugan SA. Musculoskeletal disorders of pregnancy, delivery and postpartum. Phys Med Rehabil Clin N Am 2007;18:459–76.

2. Ritchie JR. Orthopedic considerations during pregnancy. Clin Obstet Gynecol 2003;46:456–66.

3. Kristiansson P, Svardsudd K, von Schoultz B. Serum relaxin, symphyseal pain and back pain during pregnancy. Am J Obstet Gynecol 1996;175(5):1342–7.

4. Marnach M, Ramin KD, Ramsey PS, et al. Characterization of the relationship between joint laxity and maternal hormones in pregnancy. Obstet Gynecol 2003;101:331–5.

5. Charlton WPH, Coslett-Charlton LM, Ciccotti MG. Correlation of estradiol in pregnancy and anterior cruciate ligament laxity. Clin Orthop Relat Res 2001;387: 165–70.

6. Mogren IM, Pohjanen AI. Low back pain and pelvic pain during pregnancy: prevalence and risk factors. Spine 2005;30:983–91.

7. Mogren IM. Previous physical activity decreases the risk of low back pain and pelvic pain during pregnancy. Scand J Public Health 2005;33:300–6.

8. Garshasbi A, Faghih Zadeh S. The effect of exercise on the intensity of low back pain in pregnant women. Int J Gynaecol Obstet 2005;88:271–5.

9. Smith MW, Marcus PS, Wurtz LD. Orthopedic issues in pregnancy. Obstet Gynecol Surv 2008;63(2):103–11.

10. Ostgaard HC, Andersson GB, Karlsson K. Prevalence of back pain in pregnancy. Spine 1991;16(5):549–52.

11. Garmel SH, Guzelian GA, D'Alton JG, et al. Lumbar disk disease in pregnancy. Obstet Gynecol 1997;89(5 Pt 2):821–2.

12. Heckman JD, Sassard R. Current concepts review: musculoskeletal considerations in pregnancy. J Bone Joint Surg Am 1994;76:1720–30.

13. Jain N, Sternberg LB. Symphyseal separation. Obstet Gynecol 2005;105: 1229–32.

14. Kharrazi FD, Rodgers WB, Kennedy JG, et al. Parturition-induced pelvic dislocation: a report of four cases. J Orthop Trauma 1997;11:277–81.

15. Mitra R. Osteitis condensans ilii. Rheumatol Int 2010;30(3):293–6.

16. Lam CM. Worsening back pain in pregnancy. Hong Kong Med J 2007;13(5):409.

17. Guerra JJ, Steinberg ME. Distinguishing transient osteoporosis from avascular necrosis of the hip. J Bone Joint Surg Am 1995;77:616–24.

18. Wood ML, Larson CM, Dahners LE. Late presentation of a displaced subcapital fracture of the hip in transient osteoporosis of pregnancy. J Orthop Trauma 2003; 17:582–4.

19. Aynaci O, Kerimoglu S, Ozturk C, et al. Bilateral non-traumatic acetabular and femoral neck fracture due to pregnancy-associated osteoporosis. Arch Orthop Trauma Surg 2008;128(3):313–6.

20. Arayssi TK, Tawbi HA, Usta IM, et al. Calcitonin in the treatment of transient osteoporosis of the hip. Semin Arthritis Rheum 2003;32:388–97.

21. La Montagna G, Malesci D, Tirri R, et al. Successful neridronate therapy in transient osteoporosis of the hip. Clin Rheumatol 2005;24:67–9.

22. Pellicci PM, Zolla-Pazner S, Rabhan WM, et al. Osteonecrosis of the femoral head associated with pregnancy: report of three cases. Clin Orthop 1984;185:59–63.

23. Mitchell DG, Rao VM, Dalinka MK, et al. Femoral head avascular necrosis: correlation of MR imaging, radiographic staging, radionuclide imaging, and clinical findings. Radiology 1987;162:709–15.

24. Schned ES. DeQuervain's tenosynovitis in pregnant and postpartum women. Obstet Gynecol 1986;68:411–4.

25. Avci S, Yilmaz C, Sayli U. Comparison of nonsurgical treatment measure for de Quervain's disease of pregnancy and lactation. J Hand Surg Am 2002;27:322–4.

26. Choi HJ, Lee JC, Lee YJ, et al. Prevalence and clinical features of arthralgia/arthritis in healthy pregnant women. Rheumatol Int 2008;28:1111–5.
27. Silman A, Kay A, Brennan P. Timing of pregnancy in relation to the onset of rheumatoid arthritis. Arthritis Rheum 1992;35:152–5.
28. Winton GB, Lewis CW. Dermatoses of pregnancy. J Am Acad Dermatol 1982;6:977–98.
29. Sanchez NP, Pathak MA, Sato S, et al. Melasma: a clinical, light, microscopic, ultrastructural, and immunofluorescence study. J Am Acad Dermatol 1981;4:698–710.
30. Wong RC, Willis CN. Physiologic skin changes in pregnancy. J Am Acad Dermatol 1984;10:929–40.
31. Papoutsis J, Kroumpouzos G. Dermatologic disorders of pregnancy. In: Gabbe SG, Niebyl JR, Simpson JL, editors. Obstetrics: normal and problem pregnancies. 5th edition. Philadelphia: Churchill Livingstone; 2007. p. 1178–92.
32. Requena L, Yus ES. Erythema nodosum. Dermatol Clin 2008;26:425–38.
33. Mert A, Kumbasar H, Ozaras R, et al. Erythema nodosum: an evaluation of 100 cases. Clin Exp Rheumatol 2007;25:563–70.
34. Daw E. Recurrent erythema nodosum of pregnancy. Br Med J 1971;2(5752):44.
35. Bombardieri S, Munno OD, Di Punzio C, et al. Erythema nodosum associated with pregnancy and oral contraceptives. Br Med J 1977;1(6075):1509–10.
36. Gordon MC. Maternal physiology. In: Gabbe SG, Niebyl JR, Simpson JL, editors. Obstetrics: normal and problem pregnancies. 5th edition. Philadelphia: Churchill Livingstone; 2007. p. 56–84.
37. O'Brien JR. Platelet count in normal pregnancy. J Clin Pathol 1976;29:174.
38. Burrows R, Kelton J. Incidentally detected thrombocytopenia in healthy mothers and their infants. N Engl J Med 1988;319:142–5.
39. Toglia MR, Weg JG. Venous thromboembolism during pregnancy. N Engl J Med 1996;335:107–14.
40. Samuels P. Hematologic complications of pregnancy. In: Gabbe SG, Niebyl JR, Simpson JL, editors. Obstetrics: normal and problem pregnancies. 5th edition. Philadelphia: Churchill Livingstone; 2007. p. 1044–63.
41. Samuels P, Bussel JB, Braitman LE, et al. Estimation of the risk of thrombocytopenia in the offspring of pregnant women with presumed immune thrombocytopenic purpura. N Engl J Med 1990;323:229–35.
42. Terrell DR, Williams LA, Vesely SK, et al. The incidence of thrombocytopenic purpura-hemolytic uremic syndrome: all patients, idiopathic patients and patients with severe ADAMTS-13 deficiency. J Thromb Haemost 2005;3:1432–6.
43. Weiner CP. Thrombotic microangiopathy in pregnancy and the postpartum period. Semin Hematol 1987;24:119–29.
44. Sibai BM. Diagnosis, controversies, and management of the syndrome of hemolysis, elevated liver enzymes, and low platelet count. Obstet Gynecol 2004;103:981–91.
45. Sibai MB, Ramadan MK, Usta I, et al. Maternal morbidity and mortality in 442 pregnancies with hemolysis, elevated liver enzymes, and low platelets (HELLP syndrome). Am J Obstet Gynecol 1993;169:1000–6.
46. Tsirigotis P. Antiphospholipid syndrome: a predisposing factor for early onset HELLP syndrome. Rheumatol Int 2007;28(2):171–4.
47. Le Thi Thuong D, Tieulie N, Costedoat N, et al. The HELLP syndrome in the antiphospholipid syndrome: retrospective study of 16 cases in 15 women. Ann Rheum Dis 2005;64:273–8.
48. Van Oppen A, Stigter R, Bruinse H. Cardiac output in normal pregnancy: a critical review. Obstet Gynecol 1996;87:310.

49. Cutforth R, MacDonald C. Heart sounds and murmurs in pregnancy. Am Heart J 1966;71:741–7.
50. Barton JR, O'Brien JM, Bergauer NK, et al. Mild gestational hypertension remote from term: progression and outcome. Am J Obstet Gynecol 2001;184:979–83.
51. Saudan P, Brown MA, Buddle ML, et al. Does gestational hypertension become preeclampsia? BJOG 1998;105(11):1177–84.
52. Heider A, Kuller J, Strauss R, et al. Peripartum cardiomyopathy: a review of the literature. Obstet Gynecol Surv 1999;54(8):526–31.
53. Elkayam U, Akhter MW, Singh H, et al. Pregnancy-associated cardiomyopathy: clinical characteristics and a comparison between early and late presentation. Circulation 2005;111:2050–5.
54. Higby K, Suiter C, Phelps J, et al. Normal values of urinary albumin and total protein excretion during pregnancy. Am J Obstet Gynecol 1994;171:984–9.
55. Gordon M, Landon MB, Samuels P, et al. Perinatal outcome and long-term follow-up associated with modern management of diabetic nephropathy. Obstet Gynecol 1996;87:401–9.
56. Stehman-Breen C, Levine RJ, Qian C, et al. Increased risk of preeclampsia among nulliparous pregnant women with idiopathic hematuria. Am J Obstet Gynecol 2002;187:703–8.
57. Sibai BM. Diagnosis and management of gestational hypertension and preeclampsia. Obstet Gynecol 2003;102:181–92.
58. Owen J, Hauth JC. Polyarteritis nodosa in pregnancy: a case report and brief literature review. Am J Obstet Gynecol 1989;160:606–7.
59. Ekman-Ordeberg G, Sälgeback S, Ordeberg G. Carpal tunnel syndrome in pregnancy: a prospective study. Acta Obstet Gynecol Scand 1987;66:233–5.
60. Wand JS. Carpal tunnel syndrome in pregnancy and lactation. J Hand Surg 1990; 15:93–5.
61. Mondelli M. Long term follow-up of carpal tunnel syndrome during pregnancy: a cohort study and review of the literature. Electromyogr Clin Neurophysiol 2007;47(6):259–71.
62. Dike GL. Chorea gravidarum: a case report and review. Md Med J 1997;46(8): 436–9.
63. Karageyim AY, Kars B, Dansuk R, et al. Chorea gravidarum: a case report. J Matern Fetal Neonatal Med 2002;12(5):353–4.
64. Orzechowski NM, Wolanskyj AP, Ahlskog JE, et al. Antiphospholipid antibody-associated chorea. J Rheumatol 2008;35:2165–70.
65. Sibai BM. Diagnosis, prevention, and management of eclampsia. Obstet Gynecol 2005;105:402–10.
66. Chames MC, Livingston JC, Ivester TS, et al. Late postpartum eclampsia: a preventable disease? Am J Obstet Gynecol 2002;186:1174–7.
67. Bonapace E, Fisher R. Constipation and diarrhea in pregnancy. Gastroenterol Clin North Am 1998;27:197–211.

Index

Note: Page numbers of article titles are in **boldface** type.

Rheum Dis Clin N Am 36 (2010) 741–750
doi:10.1016/S0889-857X(10)00088-8
0889-857X/10/$ – see front matter © 2010 Elsevier Inc. All rights reserved.

rheumatic.theclinics.com

Moving?

Make sure your subscription moves with you!

To notify us of your new address, find your **Clinics Account Number** (located on your mailing label above your name), and contact customer service at:

Email: journalscustomerservice-usa@elsevier.com

800-654-2452 (subscribers in the U.S. & Canada)
314-447-8871 (subscribers outside of the U.S. & Canada)

Fax number: 314-447-8029

Elsevier Health Sciences Division
Subscription Customer Service
3251 Riverport Lane
Maryland Heights, MO 63043

*To ensure uninterrupted delivery of your subscription, please notify us at least 4 weeks in advance of move.

United States Postal Service

Statement of Ownership, Management, and Circulation
(All Periodicals Publications Except Requestor Publications)

1. Publication Title	2. Publication Number	3. Filing Date
Rheumatic Disease Clinics of North America	0 0 6 - 2 7 7 2	9/15/10

4. Issue Frequency	5. Number of Issues Published Annually	6. Annual Subscription Price
Feb, May, Aug, Nov	4	$264.00

7. Complete Mailing Address of Known Office of Publication (Not printer) (Street, city, county, state, and ZIP+4®)

Elsevier Inc.
360 Park Avenue South
New York, NY 10010-1710

Contact Person

Stephen Bushing

Telephone (Include area code)

215-239-3688

8. Complete Mailing Address of Headquarters or General Business Office of Publisher (Not printer)

Elsevier Inc., 360 Park Avenue South, New York, NY 10010-1710

9. Full Names and Complete Mailing Addresses of Publisher, Editor, and Managing Editor (Do not leave blank)

Publisher (Name and complete mailing address)

Kim Murphy, Elsevier, Inc., 1600 John F. Kennedy Blvd. Suite 1800, Philadelphia, PA 19103-2899

Editor (Name and complete mailing address)

Rachel Glover, Elsevier, Inc., 1600 John F. Kennedy Blvd. Suite 1800, Philadelphia, PA 19103-2899

Managing Editor (Name and complete mailing address)

Catherine Bewick, Elsevier, Inc., 1600 John F. Kennedy Blvd. Suite 1800, Philadelphia, PA 19103-2899

10. Owner (Do not leave blank. If the publication is owned by a corporation, give the name and address of the corporation immediately followed by the names and addresses of all stockholders owning or holding 1 percent or more of the total amount of stock. If not owned by a corporation, give the names and addresses of the individual owners. If owned by a partnership or other unincorporated firm, give its name and address as well as those of each individual owner. If the publication is published by a nonprofit organization, give its name and address.)

Full Name	Complete Mailing Address
Wholly owned subsidiary of	4520 East-West Highway
Reed/Elsevier, US holdings	Bethesda, MD 20814

11. Known Bondholders, Mortgagees, and Other Security Holders Owning or Holding 1 Percent or More of Total Amount of Bonds, Mortgages, or Other Securities. If none, check box ☐ None

Full Name	Complete Mailing Address
N/A	

12. Tax Status (For completion by nonprofit organizations authorized to mail at nonprofit rates) (Check one)
The purpose, function, and nonprofit status of this organization and the exempt status for federal income tax purposes:
☐ Has Not Changed During Preceding 12 Months
☐ Has Changed During Preceding 12 Months (Publisher must submit explanation of change with this statement)

PS Form 3526, September 2007 (Page 1 of 3 (Instructions Page 3)) PSN 7530-01-000-9931 PRIVACY NOTICE: See our Privacy policy in www.usps.com

---

13. Publication Title	14. Issue Date for Circulation Data Below
Rheumatic Disease Clinics of North America	August 2010

15. Extent and Nature of Circulation		Average No. Copies Each Issue During Preceding 12 Months	No. Copies of Single Issue Published Nearest to Filing Date
a. Total Number of Copies (Net press run)		1529	1380
b. Paid Circulation (By Mail and Outside the Mail)	(1) Mailed Outside-County Paid Subscriptions Stated on PS Form 3541. (Include paid distribution above nominal rate, advertiser's proof copies, and exchange copies)	574	509
	(2) Mailed In-County Paid Subscriptions Stated on PS Form 3541 (Include paid distribution above nominal rate, advertiser's proof copies, and exchange copies)		
	(3) Paid Distribution Outside the Mails Including Sales Through Dealers and Carriers, Street Vendors, Counter Sales, and Other Paid Distribution Outside USPS®	385	350
	(4) Paid Distribution by Other Classes Mailed Through the USPS (e.g. First-Class Mail®)		
c. Total Paid Distribution (Sum of 15b (1), (2), (3), and (4))	▶	959	859
d. Free or Nominal Rate Distribution (By Mail and Outside the Mail)	(1) Free or Nominal Rate Outside-County Copies Included on PS Form 3541	85	75
	(2) Free or Nominal Rate In-County Copies Included on PS Form 3541		
	(3) Free or Nominal Rate Copies Mailed at Other Classes Through the USPS (e.g. First-Class Mail)		
	(4) Free or Nominal Rate Distribution Outside the Mail (Carriers or other means)		
e. Total Free or Nominal Rate Distribution (Sum of 15d (1), (2), (3) and (4))	▶	85	75
f. Total Distribution (Sum of 15c and 15e)	▶	1044	934
g. Copies not Distributed (See instructions to publishers #4 (page 83))	▶	485	446
h. Total (Sum of 15f and g)	▶	1529	1380
i. Percent Paid (15c divided by 15f times 100)	▶	91.86%	91.97%

16. Publication of Statement of Ownership

If the publication is a general publication, publication of this statement is required. Will be printed in the November 2010 issue of this publication. ☐ Publication not required

17. Signature and Title of Editor, Publisher, Business Manager, or Owner

Stephen R. Bushing Date: September 15, 2010

Stephen R. Bushing – Fulfillment/Inventory Specialist

I certify that all information furnished on this form is true and complete. I understand that anyone who furnishes false or misleading information on this form or who omits material or information requested on the form may be subject to criminal sanctions (including fines and imprisonment) and/or civil sanctions (including civil penalties).

PS Form 3526, September 2007 (Page 2 of 3)

Printed and bound by CPI Group (UK) Ltd, Croydon, CR0 4YY

03/10/2024

01040447-0011